Autism

BREAKING THROUGH TO DISCOVER THE EXTRAORDINARY

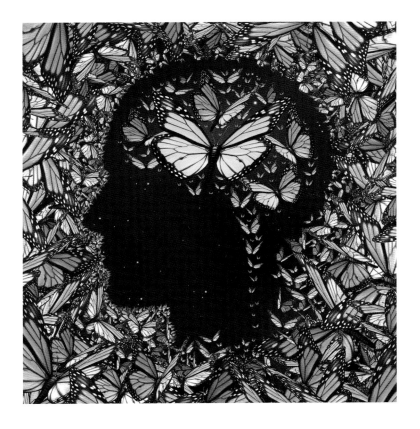

Bronwyn Davis

ABOUT THE AUTHOR

Bronwyn Davis lives in a small town in Australia's Gippsland region with her partner Jason and three young children, Aislinn, Jasper and Reilly. Although never officially diagnosed with Asperger's, she has lived with this neuro-divergence all her life and, upon receiving a diagnosis for her daughter in 2010, commenced a not-for-profit organisation known as SAAIF – 'Support & Advocacy for Autism Spectrum Individuals & Families'. Bronwyn also works as a freelance property and finance journalist and while she has regrettably had to wind down operations with the SAAIF organisation due to Reilly's recent diagnosis of Type 1 Diabetes, she continues to advocate for the Autism community and assist those on the Spectrum whenever possible. You can connect with Bronwyn and read more about embracing and nurturing your child's own 'Autistic' difference via Facebook at facebook.com/theautismbook (The Autism Book All About Different).

Published by:
Wilkinson Publishing Pty Ltd
ACN 006 042 173
Level 4, 2 Collins St Melbourne,
Victoria, Australia 3000
Ph: +61 3 9654 5446
www.wilkinsonpublishing.com

International distribution by Pineapple Media Limited
(www.pineapple-media.com) ISSN 2203-0840

Design: Spike Creative www.spikecreative.com.au

Printed in China.

National Library of Australia Cataloguing-in-Publication entry

Creator:–   Davis, Bronwyn, author.

Title: Autism : breaking through to discover the extraordinary / Bronwyn Davis.

ISBN: 9781925265095 (paperback)

Series: WP Healthy eating series.

Subjects: Autism--Australia.
                   Autism in children--Australia.
                   Parents of autistic children--Anecdotes.

Dewey Number: 618.9285882

ACKNOWLEDGEMENTS

Firstly, I would like to thank my publisher and dear friend Michael Wilkinson, for believing in the value of this book and supporting me with kindness and patience, throughout what has been a long and occasionally confronting writing process.

Thank you to my partner Jason, who has encouraged me along this journey and always accepted me for who I am, irrespective of how difficult I can be to live with at times!

Much love to my brother Tai Isa, who was the first person to really open my eyes to the truth of myself, and life in general, all those years ago in another lifetime when I struggled with my identity.

I must also acknowledge Kylie Russell for coming on the SAAIF roller coaster with me and Jackie Cheung, a woman whose genius has inspired me and whose unwavering faith kept me going when times were tough. Thanks for standing by me ladies.

Finally, a big thank you to all of the wonderful families I've met and friends I've made over the last four or so years. There is so much love, acceptance and warmth in the Autism community; I feel blessed to be a part of your difference.

I would like to dedicate this book to my beautiful children, whom I love more than anything – I'm so thankful you are your own unique selves and I hope you grow up to appreciate the incredible people you are. And to my beautiful mother Lorraine and my late father, Brian Davis, who was the first person to accept Aislinn for who she is and who encouraged my love of words and writing from a very young age. Your memory lives on in your children and grandchildren, whom you loved dearly and who will forever hold you in our hearts.

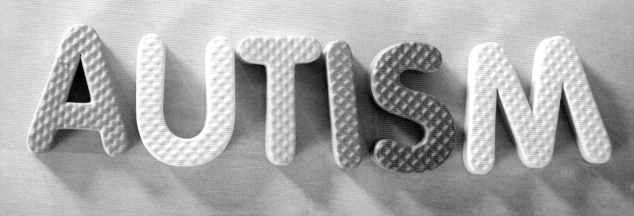

CONTENTS

CONTENTS

CHAPTER 1

WHY THIS BOOK IS (ALL ABOUT) DIFFERENT

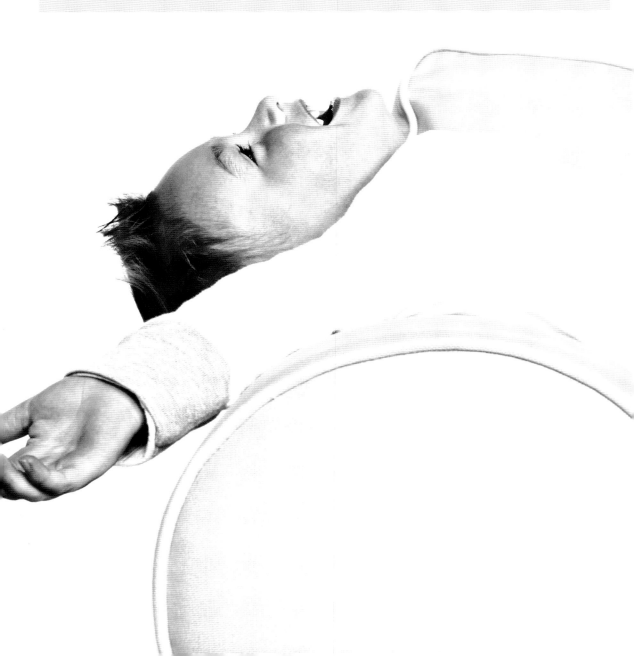

I don't profess to be a technical expert on Autism. However, this book isn't intended as a textbook guide to Autism or the Autistic person in your life.

This book isn't overflowing with references to standard descriptors of Autism – the commonly pathologised lists of behavioural, social and functional "impairments" that pervade the Autistic definition and identity.

That's because for me, this book is personal. It's inspired by and created from my own intimate insight into Autism's infinite spectrum of difference, and the experience of neuro-diversity in a world that celebrates sameness.

I have Asperger's. My brother was diagnosed in his late 30s, my 6-year-old daughter was assessed as having Asperger's and an anxiety disorder at the age of 2, my 4-year-old boy has Autism and my 3 year old exhibits numerous Autistic traits.

So it's in my own best interests to write something that deviates from the vast majority of information currently available around Autism.

Information rooted in pathologising language, which seeks to explain away as a social disorder what is essentially a person's complex experience of neural diversity.

This is harmful, destructive dialogue that has the potential to create a self-fulfilling outlook of low self-worth and restricted life outcomes among Autistic people.

In truth, Autism isn't "the problem". Nor do I believe being Autistic is intrinsically linked with having low self-esteem, or multiple impairments that render us incapable of contributing to the world in a positive, meaningful way.

To me, many of the complex issues that accompany Autism lie in a misguided stigma of what it means to be Autistic in our world, and a consistent focus on what Autistic people can't do rather than what they can do.

From the very beginning, when a child is first assessed, families are asked to define their character according to limitations and weaknesses. Invariably that imbalanced reflection of our tiny charges continues as they mature, and their needs and the needs of the family change and we attempt to access different services and supports.

As soon as the word Autism is uttered, parents go into mourning for the loss of the child they had so many expectations of.

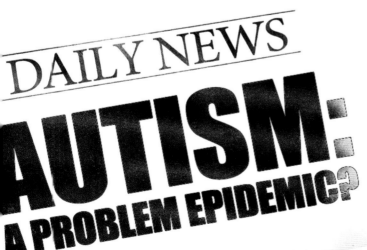

Often they're exposed to reams of information that tells them their child has little or no chance of having a productive, fulfilling life. Unless of course, they can "learn to be like everyone else."

Many parents I have spoken with share stories of the paediatrician's painfully bleak prognosis that renders their child incapable of ever learning, developing, socialising, being gainfully employed or independent, or having a family of their own someday.

It's little wonder this unproductive, problem-centric dialogue sends families into self-perpetuating spirals of frustration, hurt, helplessness and misdirection.

This book doesn't focus on or promote harmful stigmas that threaten to attach themselves to the Autistic child and follow them into adulthood.

Rather, it's based on my personal insights and musings, or on information I've encountered over years of research that resonates with my core belief - the human experience should be a journey undertaken within the natural supports of community that nurtures potential and possibility, free from a limitation bias.

Hence, this book doesn't get bogged down in the pathology of Autism as a "disease" or "disorder". It speaks to the heart and soul of Autism – as a form of neurodiversity that challenges the narrow confines of 'normal' in our world.

And it borrows most of its information from the best Autism experts I have ever spoken with – the Autistic community itself.

I hope my words (agonised over long and hard) add to the growing discourse within our community around the importance of each Autistic person's own journey of self-discovery, in an environment of support and acceptance. And that all who read this book are compelled to add their voice to this important dialogue for future generations.

I hope that you find these insights useful and derive some comfort, optimism, joy, laughter and "a-ha" moments of strength and inspiration from the journey I share with you… albeit in its abridged version.

Ultimately, this book, as with the Autistic journey itself, will mean something different to each reader. I truly hope you enjoy…

WHY AUTISM BRINGS OUT THE EXTRAORDINARY

Why do I refer to Autism as "extraordinary"? Because I see Autism as something we can learn and grow from as human beings. It makes the world a more colourful place and invites us to look beyond the limitations of 'normal'. It compels us to not only think outside "the box", but to do away with it entirely and open ourselves up to new possibilities.

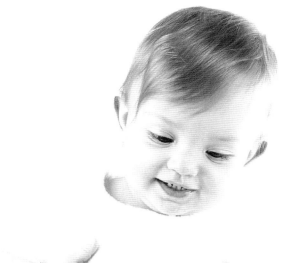
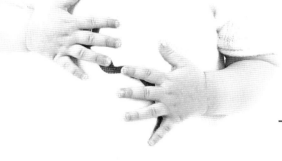
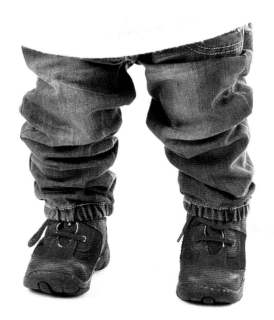

The human experience should be a journey undertaken within the natural supports of community that nurtures potential and possibility, free from a limitation bias

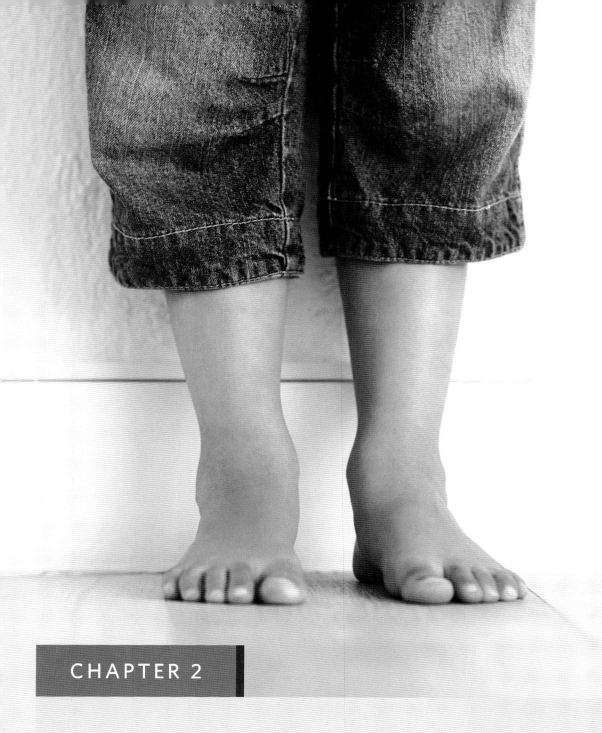

CHAPTER 2

HOW IS **AUTISM DEFINED?**

The World Health Organisation classifies Autism as a "pervasive developmental disorder." It falls under the wide-ranging "developmental disorders" banner - a group of conditions with onset in infancy or childhood.

Characterised by impairment or delay in functions related to the maturation of the central nervous system, these so-called disorders can impact a single aspect of the child's development (such as speech and language, learning and/or motor function), or several (pervasive developmental disorders and intellectual disability).

According to an article entitled '*How the Brain thinks in Autism: Implications for language intervention*', by Minshew & Williams, Autism isn't a behavioural and social communication impairment in itself, rather it's a broad-based neurodevelopmental or brain-based divergence resulting from genetic events that occur prior to birth, with widespread effects on cognitive and socio-emotional development.

At least that's the pathologised version of Autism. The nuances of Autism are intricate and complex, with virtually every Autistic person presenting with different characteristics and importantly, life experiences. Like snowflakes, no two 'Autistic patterns' are ever identical.

While all the current and historical evidence points to Autism as a form of human neurodiversity, the Autistic mind has been systematically pathologised since it was first officially recognised in the early 1900s.

Much of the negative, 'deficiency'

terminology used to classify Autistic diversity as some kind of disease, has caused the unjust stigmatization and marginalization of people who are neurally distinct for generations. Unless we stop pathologising Autism, I fear these indignities will continue.

EMPOWERING AUTISTIC PEOPLE BY DISEMPOWERING AUTISTIC DEFINITION

In 1980, the American Psychiatric Association (APA) added Autism to its widely used Diagnostic Statistical Manual (DSM). In 1994, they revised the manual to include a group of four 'Autism Spectrum Disorders', characterised by a distinct set of traits, including Autistic Disorder, Asperger Syndrome, Childhood Disintegrative Disorder and the 'catch-all' favourite, Pervasive Developmental Disorder-Not Otherwise Specified (PDD-NOS).

In May 2013, a new version of the DSM introduced yet another Autism taxonomy into the mix, after researchers found that these distinct classifications were not being applied consistently across medical practices and professionals.

Part of the issue with Autism assessment is that it's generally multi-disciplinary, involving more than one specialist, and often quite subjective in its reliance on secondhand accounts of the patient's experiences. There is no one standard scientific methodology that can determine Autism or measure its impact on the individual at this stage.

In the new DSM-5, Asperger Syndrome doesn't even rate a mention, making way for criteria that experts suggest better reflects today's knowledge of Autism, whilst providing a more accurate and medically relevant means of assessing patients.

However, I'm one of the many critics who suggest that Autism has no place at all in a diagnostic manual intended to assess mental illness. Must we identify Autistic people in the context of 'disorder', just so they can access the necessary supports to effectively manage any disabilities associated with their Autistic difference, as a social minority?

DEFICIENCIES OF THE DSM

The inclusion of Autism in the psychiatric fraternity's DSM is misleading. While those who study it still know little about Autism, there's overwhelming evidence to prove that Autism is a form of human neurodiversity; it's a mental variance. Think of the Autistic mind as having modified hard wiring.

Pathologising Autism as an illness, when it's clearly something else entirely, is a misrepresentation of our community. It simply shouldn't be happening in today's modern world, where buzzwords like 'social diversity' are bandied around freely.

Why has this marginalization of Autistic people been allowed to continue for so long? Probably for the same reason that more and more people who appear 'different' in any way are having labels forced on them with restrictive definitions – because as a society, we seek to maintain control. And we fear that which we do not understand, because we may not be able to control it.

Many suggest Autism has become a modern-day social epidemic. I would argue that the epidemic is 'Normality', and a resultant pathological fear of anything or anyone that challenges our cultural designs of 'normal'.

Over the past decade or so, there has been a distinct rise in the diagnosis of anyone who fails to willingly obey the social constructs of the day. New childhood developmental 'disorders' are being diagnosed with alarming frequency, classroom behaviours that deviate from compliance are labelled disruptive and children are branded with things like Oppositional Defiance Disorder (ODD).

If so many of our children are 'broken', as these pathologised labels would have us believe, then we need to ask ourselves; what is happening to our genetic evolution as a species? Has our DNA been so altered in the last 100 or so years of human history to justify an alleged increased incidence of 'atypical' human minds?

Or…what if we have such restricted and imposing cultural and social constructs of 'normal' human behaviour, that it's difficult not to be considered 'different'?

Is it a coincidence that the more 'normal' the world expects from us, the

What if, just what if, I'm not broken and there's nothing to fix?

UNKNOWN

more neurological divergence we are seeing in the human race?

I know this is starting to get a little socio-political, so I will refrain from going too far down this particular rabbit hole (for now). But to understand what Autism is, you must first recognise what it's not – it's not a mental illness, nor is it a psychiatric 'disorder'.

HOW THE DSM DEFINES AUTISM

The DSM-5, used by paediatricians, psychologists and psychiatrists, lists various signs and symptoms of Autism and calls for a certain number of these to be present in early childhood (even if not acknowledged until later in the person's life), before a diagnosis of 'Autism Spectrum Disorder' is applied.

These 'symptoms' are explored in the framework of two areas of difficulty. Based on how much the child (or adult being diagnosed retrospectively) is perceived to struggle in these areas, a severity ranking is applied. This is to assist in determining the level of support (and intervention) the person might require in their lifetime.

The two new areas of focus under the DSM-5 are:

1. Social and communication – recognised signs include;

- rarely speaking to others or not speaking at all
- responding inappropriately or not at all
- misreading non-verbal interactions
- having difficulty forming and maintaining age-appropriate friendships

2. Fixated interests and repetitive behaviour – examples include;

- displaying very narrow and intense interests and areas of focus
- lining toys up in a particular way over and over again

Under DSM-5 guidelines, Autism symptoms are ranked according to how prominent and consistent they appear to be in the patient, with a mild classification at Number 1 suggesting the person requires less intensive assistance, whereas a Number 3 ranking signals the need for more comprehensive support.

However, the problem with simplifying Autism down to a list of common symptoms is that the Autistic experience is anything but common.

FRUIT SALADS

One of the better ways of explaining Autism comes from a fellow Autistic woman whom I've had the pleasure of meeting, Donna Williams.

Donna was assessed as being psychotic at the age of two years. She is now a celebrated Autism consultant and educator, having published a number of books on the subject and her own life experiences.

Her work with hundreds of children since 1997 led her to conclude that Autism isn't one condition, meaning a one-size-fits-all approach to the Autistic experience and Autistic person's needs is futile.

Donna suggests that each person has their own inherent "fruit salad" of different physical, mental and emotional characteristics, and depending on the combination of these traits, the person's development and responses to the world around them will present as an 'Autistic pattern'.

She says the acknowledgement, understanding and subsequent way in which a person's "fruit salad' is "respectfully managed" will ultimately determine his or her abilities and progress as they journey through life.

This is a much more sympathetic and authentic representation of Autism than anything that's appeared in a manual penned by psychiatrists who, let's face it, are prone to view people through a restricted lens of 'normal' human behaviour.

You can read more about Donna Williams' fruit salad model of Autism on her blog – *donnawilliams.net* – and I encourage you to do so.

PROBLEMS WITH PATHOLOGISING LANGUAGE

Pathologising Autism might be convenient for medical experts and faceless corporations who control healthcare based on their bottom line rather than patient wellbeing – giving them leave to 'treat' Autism with expensive drugs and therapies. But it's in no way logical or effective.

I personally find it difficult to swallow the DSM's definition of Autism without a healthy dose of skepticism, given that the manual earns the APA over $5million in revenue every year from expensive copyright protection.

Then of course there are the ongoing issues raised by the publication's many critics, who claim it relies on superficial symptoms and artificial dividing lines between categories of dysfunction and 'normality', as well as possible cultural bias and the "medicalisation of human distress".

Let's not overlook the fact that the DSM listed 'homosexuality' as a disease up until 1974, justifying its inclusion as a supposed underlying, pathological fear of the opposite sex, with parents blamed for 'turning their children gay' through traumatic parent-child relationships.

Reducing Autism down to a narrow list of symptoms, and suggesting that in addressing these apparent issues we can 'fix' a person back to 'normal', fails to account for the many variances of each Autistic person and indeed, of humanity.

Only when we acknowledge a person's entire self and their unique "fruit salad", will we be able to nurture them through life successfully.

THE MORE 'NORMAL' WE EXPECT, THE MORE AUTISM WE SEE

According to the World Health Organisation (WHO), 1 in 160 or more than 7.6 million global citizens have Autism. It's believed however, that this figure does not accurately reflect reality, with many individuals thought to go undiagnosed in developing countries due to various cultural, social and economic constraints.

Prevalence rates in Australia (2012 - Australian Bureau of Statistics) showed an estimated 115,400 Australians, or 0.5% have Autism. This represents a 79% increase from 2009, when approximately 64,400 people were said to be on the Spectrum.

However most medical experts and academics claim this is far too conservative and that anecdotally, the reality is closer to 1 in 100.

At time of writing, the Centre for Disease Control in the US released figures collected via the Autism Developmental Disabilities Monitoring Network (ADDM), showing 1 in 68 American children are currently diagnosed with Autism, compared with 1 in 88 in 2008 and 1 in 110 in 2006. Interestingly, the CDC suggests that 45 years ago the US estimate was 20 to 30 times lower.

Canada's Autism prevalence rates are comparable to the US at 1 in 68, while in the UK about 1.1% of the population is said to be Autistic. A study on Autism in South Korea proposed that 2.64% of local children aged between seven and twelve years have some form of ASD.

Overall, the CDC and other developed nations report that the incidence of Autism is on the rise, with diagnostic rates increasing significantly over the last two decades (as illustrated in the following table from the CDC that shows the increase in America between 2000 and 2010). Many experts believe this is due to a better understanding of Autism and related signs and symptoms.

IDENTIFIED PREVALENCE OF AUTISM SPECTRUM DISORDER
ADDM Network 2000-2010 – Combining Data from All Sites

Surveillance Year	Birth Year	Number of ADDM Sites Reporting	Prevalence per 1,000 Children (range)	This is about 1 in X children...
2000	1992	6	6.7 (4.5-9.9)	1 in 150
2002	1994	14	6.6 (3.3-10.8)	1 in 150
2004	1996	8	8.0 (4.8-9.3)	1 in 125
2006	1998	11	9.0 (4.1-12.1)	1 in 110
2008	2000	14	11.3 (4.8-21.2)	1 in 88
2010	2002	11	14.7 (14.3-15.1)	1 in 68

Source: Centre for Disease Control USA

Others however, suggest that so-called 'developmental' and 'social' disorders, like Autism, are being aggressively over-diagnosed as our expectation of what 'normal' human function should look like becomes increasingly restricted, within very specific parameters of compliant behaviour.

Although it pains me to witness the constant debate surrounding the truth to these statistics, I understand society's apparent need to play down the rising number of children presenting with Autism characteristics.

Why wouldn't we want to refute a different way of processing the world when we are convinced, by the rhetoric surrounding Autism, that it's a costly and burdensome global epidemic?

WHAT CAUSES AUTISM?

Autism isn't a contagious disease contracted like the common cold. And to be honest, I haven't yet read any research findings that are convincing in their conjecture around the alleged 'risk factors' and 'causes'.

While academics and scientists have presented various hypotheses based on their preferred area of research – genetics, in-utero (pregnancy) complications or influences, environmental toxins, the divisive speculation around vaccines and mind-gut associations, to name a few - no one has come up with one conclusive answer.

There have been some very compelling studies where children who seem to develop according to 'normal' milestones until about the age of 4 years, before suddenly regressing and losing the ability to communicate or connect with those around them, are thought to become Autistic due to physiological changes.

This type of research is widely referred to as bio-medicine and suggests that the young child's exposure to certain foods, toxins, medications or other chemicals can change the highly delicate flora found in our stomach and intestine. This theory is based on a belief that our brain function is directly linked to the health of our gut and any serious imbalance can trigger developmental disruptions.

I know from my own experience, and that of my children, how important diet and lifestyle can be in managing things like anxiety, fatigue, behavioural triggers and overall mental health, so this is an area I find fascinating.

However, the notion that diet alone can 'cause' someone to become Autistic is one I find difficult to swallow. Could exposure to certain biological allergens or toxins potentially replicate the pathologised descriptors of Autism? I have no doubt this is possible.

Just as it's possible that certain trauma experiences, which occur throughout a child's development, can trigger behaviours that mimic Autistic patterns. But Autism in itself is a human neurological divergence.

In the late 1940s, Bruno Bettelheim laid the blame for Autism squarely at the feet of cold, unfeeling parents when he coined the term "refrigerator mothers".

This guilt-laden theory stuck for many years and even now, parents often question whether they have done something (or failed to do something) to create their child's Autism.

Given that Autism is often present among multiple members of the same family bloodlines, it's now widely agreed among the scientific community that certain genetic dynamics and predispositions play a major role in the evolution of this particular neurodiversity.

WHY WE NEED A COMPLETE RETHINK ON AUTISM

Much of the dialogue around Autism – in professional circles, the increasingly profitable global Autism industry and even in the community itself – is embedded in a pathologised perception of the Autistic person as being 'unwell' or 'broken' in some way.

Living in our own skin isn't enough. We are coerced to change and 'fit in'. This is particularly obvious when discussion around early detection of Autism in children is based on how quickly and effectively 'treatment' can occur to 'intervene' with the Autistic journey.

AUTISM STATS FROM THE CDC – "RISK FACTORS"

- Studies have shown that among identical twins, if one child has ASD, then the other will be affected about 36-95% of the time. In non-identical twins, if one child has ASD, then the other is affected about 0-31% of the time.

- Parents who have a child with ASD have a 2%–18% chance of having a second child who is also affected.

- ASD tends to occur more often in people who have certain genetic or chromosomal conditions. About 10% of children with Autism are also identified as having Down syndrome, fragile X syndrome, tuberous sclerosis, or other genetic and chromosomal disorders.

- Children born to older parents are at a higher risk for having ASD.

- A small percentage of children who are born prematurely or with low birth weight are at greater risk for having ASD.

- ASD commonly co-occurs with other developmental, psychiatric, neurologic, chromosomal, and genetic diagnoses. The co-occurrence of one or more non-ASD developmental diagnoses is 83%. The co-occurrence of one or more psychiatric diagnoses is 10%.

Source: Centre for Disease Control USA

Even phrases that usually represent promise and potential – "optimal life outcomes" is one that comes to mind – are now used with the implication that "optimal" means "curing" the person of their Autism.

This pathology framework compels parents to understand their child within the parameters of the Autism stigma. It speaks to an expectation of incapacity that eventually starts to define and shape the direction the person's life takes.

We become reactive to 'the Autism' as a problem and forget how to interact naturally with our Autistic brothers and sisters, from a place of simple human connection.

By focusing on a list of 'symptoms' rather than a person's distinct character, we are at risk of overlooking important information that's communicated indirectly, about their experience of Autistic difference.

All Autistic quirks and behaviours are actually their own, very powerful type of language and expression. They can inform us as to a person's sensory triggers for one, and point to aspects of daily living that are most confronting and difficult to navigate.

So you see, 'difference' is a very useful language to understand if we hope to provide the right kind of supports for Autistic people to live a fulfilled life.

When we reduce life to a series of 'normal' affectations, founded on cultural and social expectations, then enforce this as the accepted state in which all of humanity should live, we do the neurodivergents among us a massive injustice.

Even traits that could positively influence learning and development outcomes in the Autistic child, when appropriately applied and directed - such as "narrow areas of focus" and "repetitive behaviours" - are automatically discussed within a negative, limitation context.

Rather than being so driven by a thirst for knowledge and natural curiosity to study something intensely and with single-minded clarity of purpose, little Johnny is 'obsessive' about trains due to his 'inflexible' imaginative process.

I believe it's time we rethink Autism, as a strong, supportive and connected community that chooses to direct its own unique path. In sharing our stories we can provide honest and direct insight into the possibilities of Autism; all it has to teach us, and the many amazing directions in which the Autistic journey of difference can lead our world.

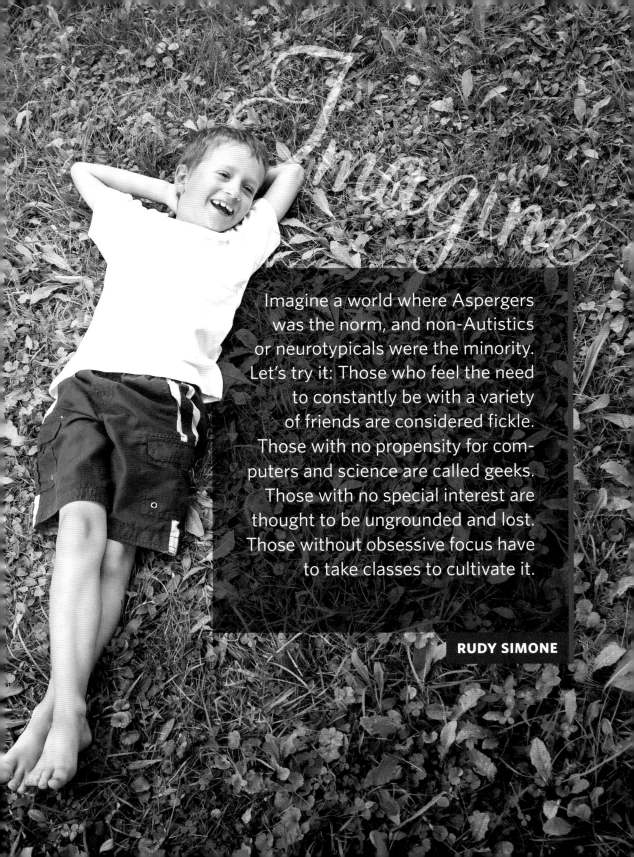

Imagine

Imagine a world where Aspergers was the norm, and non-Autistics or neurotypicals were the minority. Let's try it: Those who feel the need to constantly be with a variety of friends are considered fickle. Those with no propensity for computers and science are called geeks. Those with no special interest are thought to be ungrounded and lost. Those without obsessive focus have to take classes to cultivate it.

RUDY SIMONE

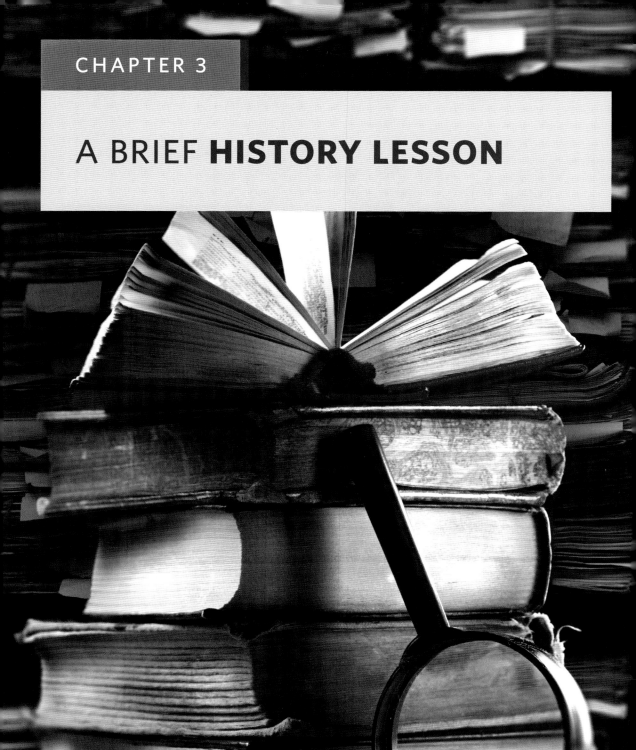

CHAPTER 3

A BRIEF **HISTORY LESSON**

Autism has a relatively short history in medical annals, with the term first used among the psychiatric fraternity in 1911 to describe a selective introverted state of 'selfism', commonly observed in schizophrenic patients.

Since the first half of the twentieth century, countless academics, scientists and mental health professionals have studied Autism voraciously, and some might suggest 'obsessively' (I know – ironic isn't it?).

Even though billions of dollars have been spent in the search for Autistic 'causes' and subsequent 'cures', there are still arguably more mysteries surrounding this vast Spectrum, than answers as to why some people experience life through the Autistic perspective.

Some experts suggest that Autism has existed since our cavemen ancestors walked the earth, and that without a peppering of Autistic traits throughout human history we would not have advanced so far along the evolutionary path.

Many discoveries that have changed the course of life, as we know it – fire, electricity and the Internet for instance – have been credited to the unique problem solving capacity exhibited by neurodivergent minds.

Today, it's widely held that notable historical figures who exhibited some form of academic or creative genius, were considered 'quirky' or 'odd', did not meet typical developmental milestones as children and failed to excel in a rigid

scholarly environment (think Einstein and Mozart), were most likely on the Autism Spectrum.

> For success in science or in art, a dash of Autism is essential. The essential ingredient may be an ability to turn away from the everyday world, from the simply practical and to rethink a subject with originality so as to create in new untrodden ways with all abilities channelled into the one specialty.

HANS ASPERGER

AUTISM AND ASPERGER'S – A HISTORICAL TIMELINE

1911 – Psychiatrist Eugen Bleuler first uses the terms 'Autism' and 'Autistic' to describe an aspect of schizophrenia observed in his patients, whereby the person socially withdraws from the world around them in a process of active detachment. 'Autism' comes from the Greek work 'autos' meaning self - i.e. Autism literally translates to 'selfism'.

1943 – American psychiatrist, Leo Kanner, stumbles across the term 'Autism' and recognises its potential application in the patients he's been treating, who he initially believed were experiencing childhood schizophrenia. Upon realising that the eleven children in his care were not exhibiting typical schizophrenic symptoms, he used the term 'Infantile Autism' to describe their condition.

Kanner published a paper on his discoveries in the UK, gaining significant attention and acclaim.

1944 - Soon after Kanner starts talking 'Autism', Austrian paediatrician Hans Asperger uses the term 'Autistic psychopathy' to describe four boys referred to his psychiatric clinic, with what presented as a personality disorder.

Asperger was one of the first to recognise that unlike schizophrenia, children with Autism did not display any personality disintegration or psychosis.

Asperger described the main 'symptoms' exhibited by the boys as lacking nonverbal communication skills, failing to demonstrate empathy with their peers and being physically clumsy.

Since his death in 1980, there's been considerable speculation as to whether Asperger himself exhibited characteristics of the 'Syndrome' as a child. He often referred to his young patients as "little professors" and believed some of them would go on to achieve exceptional success later in life.

Asperger followed the progress of one patient - Fritz V - into adulthood. His belief that these were extraordinarily capable minds was confirmed when Fritz became a professor of astronomy and solved an error in Isaac Newton's work that he first uncovered as a child.

Asperger opened what was conceivably the first specialist school for children with

THE 'KANNER 11' CHARACTERISTICS

The following is a list of traits (eleven coincidentally) that Kanner described in the eleven children he studied:

1. Inability to relate to others in an ordinary manner
2. Extreme aloneness that isolates children from the outside world
3. Apparent resistance to being picked up or held by parents
4. Deficits in language, including 'mutism' and echolalia
5. Excellent rote memory in some instances
6. Early specific food preferences
7. Extreme fear reactions to loud noises
8. Obsessive desire for repetition and maintenance of sameness
9. Few spontaneous activities, such as typical play behaviour
10. Bizarre and repetitive physical movement, such as spinning or rocking
11. Normal physical appearance

Source: *Scheuermann & Weber, 2002*

Autism, toward the end of the Second World War. A bombing razed the school before it commenced operations in earnest and much of Asperger's early work was destroyed.

Late 1940s – Hungarian Bruno Bettelheim, who claimed to be a psycho-therapist before it was revealed in the 1990s that he had no relevant degree, studies the effect of three therapy sessions with children he determined to be 'Autistic'.

He subsequently claimed their condition was due to the emotional frigidity of their mothers, from whom the young charges were removed. Kanner supported Bettelheim's theory and the pair worked towards proving their new hypothesis, which suggested 'Refrigerator Mothers' caused Autism.

1964 – American psychologist and parent of an Autistic child, Bernard Rimland (founder of the Autism Society of America), disagrees with Bettelheim's claims that parental attachment issues caused his son's Autism as an emotional illness.

He publishes '*Infantile Autism: The syndrome and its implications for a neural therapy of behaviour*', which spoke of Autism as a biological disorder.

1970s – Autism is more widely discussed, however many parents and doctors continue to mistake Autistic traits for childhood psychosis and 'mental retardation'. Sadly, it's believed thousands of children were wrongly diagnosed and placed in institutional care.

1981 – English based psychiatrist and physician Lorna Wing, who has an Autistic daughter, publishes an academic paper entitled 'Asperger's Syndrome: a Clinical Account'; popularizing Asperger's previous work along with the term 'Asperger Syndrome'.

Wing was highly influential in the UK Autism community, uniting with other parents of Autistic children in 1962 to establish the National Autistic Society (NAS), and writing a number of highly acclaimed books on the subject, including comprehensive guides for parents and teachers.

Wing and her colleague Judith Gould concluded that Autism exists on a continuum (or spectrum) after conducting a groundbreaking study in 1979. In the 1990s Wing, along with Christopher Gillberg from the Children's Neuro-Psychiatric Clinic in Sweden, found the triad of disturbed mutual contact, disturbed mutual communication and limited imagination, commonly referred to as the 'triad of impairments'.

In the 1980s they added a fourth Autistic factor of limited planning ability – more commonly known today as 'executive dysfunction'.

1989 – Gillberg & Gillberg outline sets of diagnostic criteria for Autism.

1991 – London based developmental psychiatrist Uta Frith, translates Hans Asperger's paper to English.

1992 – Asperger Syndrome becomes a standard diagnosis after it's inclusion in the tenth edition of the World Health

Organisation's, International Classification of Diseases.

1994 - Asperger Syndrome is added to the globally recognised fourth edition of the American Psychiatric Association's Diagnostic and Statistical Manual of Mental Disorders (DSM IV), distinguishing it from Autistic disorder with its own list of symptoms and characteristics.

2013 - Asperger Syndrome is removed from the revised DSM-5, eliminating it as a separate diagnosis and rolling it into the broader Autism Spectrum, based on a severity scale.

AUTISM AND ASPERGER'S HALL OF FAME

Much speculation exists as to whether a number of famous historical figures were actually Autistic, and whether their capacity for processing the world in different ways contributed to their respective life's work.

Clinicians, academics and biographers have retrospectively diagnosed a number of famous people throughout history. Although controversy surrounds claims that these people of note were on the Spectrum, it's an interesting conversation starter and an area I personally find intriguing. So let's look at some of the better-known 'Autistic' personalities of the past...

- **Stanly Kubrick** – filmmaker
- **Emily Dickinson** – poet
- **James Joyce** – Irish author
- **Michelangelo** – Italian Renaissance artist

- **Wolfgang Amadeus Mozart** – composer
- **Blind Tom Wiggins** – Autistic musical savant
- **Charles Richter** – seismologist and creator of the Richter Scale
- **Isaac Newton** - physicist and mathematician
- **Nikola Tesla** – inventor, engineer and futurist
- **Albert Einstein** – theoretical physicist

Numerous famous faces from more recent times have candidly discussed their own personal diagnosis on the Autism Spectrum. These successful men and women are influential in challenging negative and limiting social stigmas, demonstrating that Autism need not prevent a person from reaching their full life's potential. So let's take a moment to acknowledge...

FAMOUS ASPERGIANS

- **Danny Beath** – award-winning British landscape and wildlife photographer
- **Susan Boyle** – British singer and Britain's Got Talent finalist
- **Lizzy Clark** – actress and campaigner
- **Tim Ellis** – Australian magician and author
- **Daryl Hannah** – actress
- **Clay Marzo** – American professional surfer
- **Les Murray** – Australian poet
- **Ari Ne'eman** – American Autism rights activist
- **Jerry Newport** – American author and mathematical savant, basis of the film

Mozart and the Whale

- **Craig Nicholls** – frontman of the Australian alternative rock band, The Vines
- **Tim Page** – Pulitzer Prize-winning critic and author
- **Dawn Prince-Hughes** – Ph.D., primate anthropologist, ethologist, and author
- **John Elder Robison** – author of Look Me in the Eye and Raising Cubby
- **Vernon L. Smith** – Nobel Laureate in economics
- **Adam Young** – multi-instrumentalist, producer and the founder of the electronic project Owl City
- **Dan Akroyd (dec)** – actor and producer

FAMOUS AUTISTICS

- **Temple Grandin** – food animal handling systems designer and author
- **Courtney Love** – lead singer of rock band Hole
- **Caiseal Mor** – author, musician

and artist
- **Dylan Scott Pierce** – wildlife illustrator
- **Donna Williams** – author, artist, singer-songwriter and Autism consultant
- **Marty Balin** – singer/songwriter with Jefferson Airplane
- **Lucy Blackman** – university educated author
- **Christopher Knowles** – American poet
- **Jonathon Lerman** – artist
- **Matt Savage** – US jazz prodigy
- **50 Tyson** – rapper and Autism activist
- **Richard Wawro** – Scottish artist

I see people with Asperger's syndrome as a bright thread in the rich tapestry of life

TONY ATTWOOD

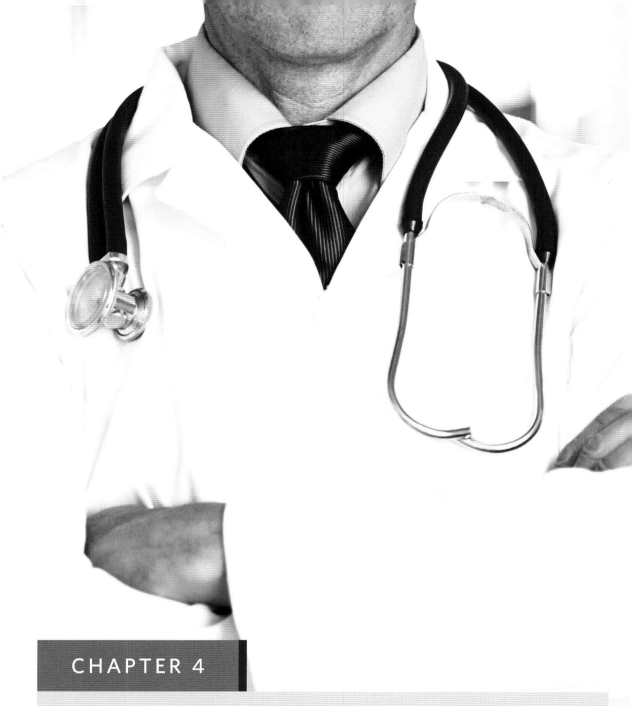

CHAPTER 4

AUTISM SIGNS AND SYMPTOMS

It's not surprising that there is so much confusion about how Autism actually presents or more importantly, feels for those who live it every day, given that Autistic people are all too often omitted from key conversations around this topic.

Autism is typically first suspected in children as a result of different social, developmental, language and communication patterns, including non-verbal communication and emotional interaction with caregivers.

These differences may represent significant 'delays', as in the case of children who don't develop speech, 'lose' their speech as toddlers or have trouble connecting with the world around them, or less pronounced distinctions.

Various atypical behaviours are also present in most instances and often there will be clear indicators of anxiety – particularly separation anxiety – and sleep disorders accompanying the experience of Autism.

Autistic behaviours can be mistakenly perceived as defiance, causing some children on the Spectrum to be wrongfully labelled as naughty, or willfully harmful, disruptive and destructive.

Autism is something the person lives with throughout their life and will experience in different ways and extremes along their personal journey.

In this chapter, I'm going to share with you some of the more commonly recognised signs and 'symptoms' of Autism, remembering that my experiences and therefore observations around this pathology definition have led me to some very different ideas about what they represent.

THE TRIAD OF IMPAIRMENTS – A PREFACE

I'm not a fan of the 'impairment' model of Autism. Certain Autistic distinctions can obviously manifest as a form of disability, however I believe many Autistic 'impairments' can actually become strengths of character for the individual who is nurtured with an understanding of their differences.

In these instances, one could argue that so-called impairments become enhancements, enriching the individuals' personality and representing a key strength of difference that can lead to successful life outcomes.

UNCOVERING THE TRIAD'S ORIGINS

History buffs who were paying attention in the last chapter will recall that Lorna Wing and Judith Gould identified the 'Triad of Impairments', after groundbreaking research in 1979.

Their studies of children with learning difficulties in a South London borough led them to conclude that certain language and communication, social and emotional and learning as well as behavioural developmental delays and differences could be "clustered together" in order to diagnose Autism in children.

This model became synonymous with assessment protocols and the 'Triad' has been applied in diagnosing and determining the 'severity' of a child's Autism for many years.

Although new diagnostic criteria has been introduced in the revised DSM-5, Gould and Wing's 'Triad' is still recognised as a foundation for determining the presence of Autism in children. So let's take a look at the three areas of 'impairment' attributed to the differences found in those on the Autism Spectrum.

1. SOCIAL INTERACTION

Depending on the type of 'socially impaired' behaviours demonstrated, children might be described as:

Aloof – Avoiding eye contact, these are the daydreamers who are said to be "in a world of their own". They may seem unresponsive when spoken to or shown affection, so it's not uncommon for this Autistic personality type to be wrongfully accused of being defiant. I like to think of these people as still waters who run deep.

Passive – This is the child who seems to "play along" with social interactions, but is assuming a passive, observer type role. I was the passive child, teenager, University student and young adult. I accepted social approaches not necessarily to partake with my peers, but to study the expectations and interactions that made my life so awkwardly anxious at times.

Active, but odd – This is my daughter to a "T"! She really wants to make friends, but just doesn't get the 'social conventions'. I find her approach to new children fascinating to watch, but I understand how it can be a little unnerving for her playground peers, who have been taught to socialise in certain 'acceptable' ways.

Active but odd types try to foster interactions by doing things like ignoring the person they really want to speak with, sometimes staring for longer than 'normal' or displaying poor eye contact, and giving overly-enthusiastic (read affectionate!) handshakes or bear-hugs.

Overly formal or stilted – I occasionally slip into this category. Autistic adults who have studied their 'neurotypical' counterparts for many years, might "act out" social interactions by being overly polite and formal, carefully following learnt social mores, and exhibiting a wide vocabulary and use of language during conversation.

On the surface, these interactions can appear 'normal', but the robotic gestures, responses and monotone speech that Autistic people with this particular social tendency can adapt tend to scream, well, different! Think Sheldon Cooper from The Big Bang Theory as the 'stilted' Autistic stereotype!

2. COMMUNICATION

Distinct differences in language and speech are often present in people with Autism. Some children develop language according to the recognised milestones or even precociously, only to regress to a state of no speech or limited/disordered speech at around 3 to 4 years of age. In some instances speech can be fully recovered and relearnt, however others never regain full speech.

Our children never 'lost speech', however they all have some very interesting variances and recognised Autistic patterns when it comes to verbal communication.

With increasing access to augmentative and assisted communication devices and apps, along with various pictorial and signing resources, we are starting to see more instances where those who remain non-verbal demonstrate remarkable insight and intelligence, when communicating through means other than speech.

Common Autistic nuances in speech and communication include:

Echolalia – repeating words and/or regurgitating scripts from favourite movies and TV shows. We affectionately call our 3 year old "the parrot".

Rote like, detailed responses to questions as though reading from a book.

Using excessive detail to explain a situation or concept – guilty!

Literal interpretation – this is a big one I have to watch out for in our household. I have learnt the great art of sarcasm and figurative speech over time, in which much of what is said isn't at all intended to be literal.

However my daughter isn't quite there yet. When I said to her the other day, "I saw that top and thought, 'That has Aislinn's name written all over it!'" She naturally responded with, "Where? I can't see it!"

Humour and sarcasm (verbal ambiguity) are often said to elude some people with Autism. I personally think I'm hilarious and laugh at lots of things. However, I have listened to so many "knock, knock" jokes from my children without any real punch line to recognise that not everyone 'gets it' at first! In my experience, learning to laugh at myself was a great way to understand humour – having an older brother also made it a necessity!

Intonation and voice control are frequent issues in our household. Commonly displayed characteristics in this area include:

- using tones and inflections inappropriately - as in the voice rising when asking a question or falling when making a statement,
- having problems adjusting volume - our daughter has an 'outside voice' wherever she goes,
- over-emphasizing words when EE-NUNN-CEE-ATE-ING and my personal favourite,
- an accent that defies the person's actual country of origin - our 4 year old is a Swiss Canadian, heralding from Ireland according to his affectations of speech.

Interpreting and applying non-verbal communication – when you are taking in every little detail of the world around you, the overload is understandably overwhelming. Staying focused on a conversation can be hard work for highly sensitive Autistic people.

All those extra non-verbal messages – eye movement, facial expressions, gestures, changes in posture and the like can easily be overlooked or misinterpreted.

> When you see an object, it seems that you see it as an entire thing first, and only afterwards do its details follow on. But for people with Autism, the details jump straight out at us first of all, and then only gradually, detail by detail, does the whole image float up into focus.

NAOKI HIGASHIDA

3. THINKING AND BEHAVIOUR

Repetitive and restricted behaviours and a seemingly reduced capacity to engage in imaginative play are commonly associated with Autism.

The little boy spinning a single wheel on the toy truck rather than driving it on imaginary roads, or the child who stacks blocks in a colour sequence instead of building a model house, are typical examples.

Experts suggest this "lack of imaginative play" prevents children from modelling human interactions and ultimately limits their empathy and understanding of other people's emotions. I disagree with pretty much all of this!

In fact if you want to see an example of restricted and repetitive behaviour in action, just look at all those alleged 'normal' people who conform to a rigid corporate identity every day for the sake of a buck!

Repetitive stereotyped activities – Examples can include spinning objects, turning lights on and off, lining toys up sequentially and collecting oddities. Some repetitive behaviour can be harmful, such as head banging and biting, particularly if the underlying cause for the so-called 'Self Injurious Behaviour' isn't adequately addressed (more on this later).

Other areas that this particular characteristic can impact include family meal and bedtime routines - with the child's need for things to be 'just so' controlling these common household activities with army like precision – and narrow areas of focus on things like numbers and weather patterns.

A SPECTRUM OF DIFFERENCES AND DISTINCTIONS

Since the introduction of revised assessment criteria for ASDs in the new DSM-5, some Autistic traits have been added and others removed in order to qualify a person for diagnosis. Characteristics required for diagnosis will be explored further in the next chapter.

For now though, it's important to note that there are many varieties of the Autistic experience and numerous combinations of traits – remember Donna William's "fruit salad" analogy?

Which is why the saying goes, "If you've met one person with Autism, you've met one person with Autism."

Additionally, as Autistic people mature and learn about the world around them (according to intellectual capacity), including various social expectations and rules, the Autistic experience will change and some things that were once 'obstacles' to social interaction can be overcome.

Then of course there are important milestones and transitions throughout the person's life that can cause an increase or decrease in the instance and/or severity of the Autistic experience. Think starting school, moving house, changes in the family dynamic, the hormonal roller coaster of adolescence, college or university and employment for instance.

Nobel prize-calibre geniuses often have certain core Autistic features at their heart.

ALLAN SNYDER,
Director of Sydney University's
Centre for the Mind.

UNDERSTANDING AUTISTIC BEHAVIOURS ACROSS THE SPECTRUM

Life on the Autism Spectrum comes with its share of personal challenges. One of the big ones is around hyper or hypo sensitivity – being extremely sensitive to touch, taste, smell, sound and sight on the one hand and on the other, seeking extra sensory input and stimulation and/or demonstrating unresponsiveness to pain.

Then there are the associated co-morbidities that can make the Autistic experience even more complex:

- anxiety,
- depression,
- sleep disturbance and irregularities,
- food aversions and 'obsessions' (some children insist only on eating foods that are white for instance),
- intellectual disability,
- learning difficulties like dyslexia and dyspraxia, and
- other health concerns, including digestive and auto-immune dysfunction, seizures and epilepsy.

This array of variables that can increase, decrease and sometimes seem to disappear or take a 360-degree turn (as happened with our daughter who went from barely responding to pain as a toddler to screaming hysterically over a paper cut), often make life on the Spectrum fairly unpredictable.

Behaviours associated with sensory issues and anxieties are common and can be confronting for parents to manage. You essentially have to throw everything you have learnt about discipline out the window with the Autistic child, because trying to address their distinct behaviours with typical punishments or reprimands alone will fail to yield positive results.

Remember, behaviours are a representation of the person's Autistic experience and a way of communicating this experience - focusing on and punishing the behaviours alone, means failing to acknowledge and properly manage the person's triggers.

> Even for parents of children that are not on the spectrum, there is no such thing as a normal child.

VIOLET STEVENS,
mum of a son with Autism

STIMMING AND AUTISM

One of the more distinct traits associated with Autism is known as stimming – a term used to describe repetitive or unusual noises or body movements made by Autistic people as self-stimulatory or soothing behaviour.

All humans 'stim' at various times and for various reasons, usually to self soothe or maintain focus and concentration – think of children who suck their thumbs or twirl their hair, adults who chew or fidget with pens to alleviate the monotony of boardroom meetings and 'leg jigglers', whose stims are often elicited by a problematic task or some anxiety trigger.

Given that Autism can represent an emotionally charged and very distinct journey in an often unforgiving and confronting world, it's not surprising that Autistic stims can occur with much greater regularity, and be more obvious and less "socially appropriate" than the stims of 'neurotypicals'.

Of course as with everything Autism, the nature of stims will vary depending on where the person sits on the Spectrum and can include:

- movements like finger flicking or hand flapping,
- rocking back and forth while sitting or standing,
- visual stims, like looking at things sideways, watching objects spinning or fingers flutter in front of the eyes,
- repetitive opening and closing of doors or turning lights on and off – we've had intermittent periods of strobe-like disco lighting effects throughout our house for the past six years now.
- chewing or mouthing – Aislinn did this until about the age of 4 and Jasper chewed on his doona every night until recently.
- Listening to the same song or noise over and over – Aislinn used to go to sleep with one of her favourite tunes playing loudly on repeat, creating many musical aversions for me in the process (there's only so many times you can hear the same Avril Lavigne or Taylor Swift song without going quietly mad!).

Another one that Aislinn used to do is humming or tongue clicking. I can often determine her mood by the frequency and tone of her vocal stims.

Research suggests that stimming occurs for a number of different reasons. For some it can be a case of seeking sensory input (for hypo-sensitive Autistic types), or trying to self soothe in the face of sensory overload by focusing all of our attention on one thing we feel in control of (the act of stimming itself).

For others it can indicate excitement or an increase in anxiety. It pays to be observant so you can gauge the subtle triggers and responses to stimming behaviours in your child.

Many of the stims and repetitive behaviours in our house are self-soothing techniques employed to level out emotional anxiety, or sensory overloads that threaten to otherwise boil over.

Stimming is another aspect of the Autistic experience that engenders considerable debate. Within a number of therapeutic approaches are interventions intended to reduce or eliminate stims, given that some stims are considered 'socially inappropriate', and at the extreme end of the Spectrum, can pose a danger to the person's wellbeing.

On the other hand, many believe stimming should be recognised as a type of 'self-management' tool for the Autistic person to draw on as required. By allowing and accepting stimming behaviour (as long as it's not causing harm to anyone), we are actually encouraging the person to achieve an intuitive self-awareness and take one step closer to independence.

MELTDOWNS VERSUS TANTRUMS – YES, THERE IS A DIFFERENCE

I'm not going to spend a massive amount of time telling you what a meltdown looks like, because if you're reading this book, chances are you've lived with and/or through your own fair share of them – so I would be preaching to the choir!

Needless to say, a meltdown isn't a tantrum, but it can be very hard to distinguish from one. It can look the same, with screaming, yelling, throwing of limbs and objects, door slamming, fists flying, kicking and biting. But the difference is in the triggers, duration, severity and most importantly, the child's ability to control these episodes.

My experience of meltdowns became more pronounced as a teenager and adult, when my emotional responses could be quite extreme.

I recall kicking a hole in the wall at the age of seventeen in response to overwhelming feelings of frustration and betrayal, when speaking with a long-time friend who had completely broken my trust. Not to mention many mornings spent cursing my reflection and throwing various hair accessories and appliances in a fit of rage over a stray hair.

I learnt as an adult, undergoing therapy for Post Natal Depression many years later, that regardless of what seemed to cause my meltdowns – bad hair days or toxic friendships – the same chemical reaction in my brain triggered all of them.

Meltdowns are a physical manifestation of the 'fight or flight response', which (long story short) causes our bodies to fuel up on adrenaline in the face of some impending danger. We experience something that excites us in a good or bad way, we react physically and the brain produces a chemical response.

That's why you can track the progression of a meltdown if you have seen them happen often enough, from the build-up and catalyst, to the onset, the escalation, the plateau and the de-escalation.

As a parent, if you observe your child's

behaviours and learn their unspoken language, you are one step closer to helping them identify their meltdown triggers, so they can better manage these episodes and reduce their frequency.

Meltdowns can be exhausting and confusing for parents, as well as the children, teenagers and adults experiencing them. But if we take meltdowns as communications of what is going on for the person at different times, they can provide valuable insight into the unique needs of the individual and allow us to learn more about the intricacies of Autistic difference.

> When living with a neurological condition (or with a loved one who has one), it can be very easy to focus on the challenges and limitations. But in my life, I have found that focusing on abilities, finding new ways to adapt, have been crucial to my successes. Seeking those solutions can even be seen as a form of creativity.

LYNNE SORAYA

DEBUNKING THE MANY AUTISM MYTHS

As mentioned at the very beginning of this chapter, I have some difficulty talking about the many 'Autistic impairments' discussed throughout these pages.

I believe a lot of Autistic traits have been incorrectly pathologised throughout the last few decades, as dialogue around Autism in our world has focused on one of two things:

1. The perceived 'problems', 'deficiencies' and social and economic costs of Autism as a health issue.
2. Scientific and academic studies in context of Autism as a disorder to be cured, rather than as a difference, with genuine consideration of the true Autistic experience.

Negative connotations are applied to the different, distinguishing characteristics of Autistic personalities, leaving very little scope (or hope) of exploring the person's possibilities and potential without being confined by limiting expectations.

Some Autistic traits paint a picture of unfeeling, withdrawn and emotionally unreachable people, failing to account for the many varied experiences of Autism in a world that misunderstands and misinterprets the intricate nuances of neurodiversity.

Here, I explore some of the more common Autism myths to demonstrate how varied the human neurodivergent Spectrum actually is and that as such, we cannot take anyone's unique Autistic journey for granted.

MYTH # 1 – ALL AUTISTIC PEOPLE ARE GIFTED OR HAVE 'SAVANT' ABILITIES

Autistic children can develop exceptional talent in one or more disciplines when their fascinations or 'passionate obsessions' are fostered with acceptance. Many will actually demonstrate where their life's path might lead as toddlers.

I often look at children who LOVE Lego and see future engineers, architects and builders. At children who adore all things railway and wonder what they might invent one day to more efficiently transport humans from one place to another, as some kind of logistics expert.

Aislinn started showing a deep interest in art and creative pursuits as soon as she could hold a pen. We have our very own five or so galleries worth of her works stored away – each one of her drawings too good not to keep.

Then there are children considered to have savant abilities, who are exceptionally gifted when it comes to things like number sequences, physics, computer language or creative pursuits such as music or art.

The belief that every Autistic individual has some kind of exceptional talent might appear to be a myth at this point in time. Many would argue that children who are seemingly incapable of speech or any form of communication, those who grow up depending on their carer just to manage daily living, aren't gifted. This is considered especially true for children who test low on conventional IQ tests.

But for me the jury is out on this one. I feel we haven't yet provided a world in which neurodiversity is effectively accepted and accommodated. We favour conformity in our education systems and as such, only provide a small scope of learning opportunities and experiences that insist on everyone acquiring knowledge and skills in the same vein, at the same pace, and around the same subjects.

All I know is that in our ideal Autistic world (where every human is nurtured and accepted within a connected and caring community), every child would have the opportunity to shine their own unique inner light to make the world a little brighter.

MYTH # 2 - PEOPLE WITH AUTISM DON'T EXPERIENCE OR SHOW EMOTIONS

Children, teenagers and adults on the Autism Spectrum feel emotions and yes, even love, although they might express these sentiments differently or have trouble understanding today's 'socially acceptable' means of emotional communication.

Given the various sensory issues Autistic people can experience, along with confusion as to the subtle undertones of non-verbal communication, we can tend to feel more comfortable when physical displays of affection are on our terms, rather than according to the expectations of others.

But don't we all feel that way about our 'personal space'? Why would someone on The Spectrum be any different in that respect?

Displays of affection are often 'normalised' within cultural and social constructs. It might not be a lingering embrace or a whispered "I love you", but trust me when I tell you that Autistic people are as capable of experiencing and expressing feelings as any other human being on the planet.

MYTH # 3 – ALL AUTISTIC PEOPLE HAVE A LEARNING DISABILITY

While Spectrum children might have difficulties in the context of 'standardised education', they can successfully acquire knowledge and/or new skills when teaching styles are properly adapted to suit their way of learning.

Research suggests that Autistic people are often better at processing information visually and /or kinetically rather than verbally. So why do we insist on integrating our children into 'mainstream schooling' that favours a verbal learning approach and ignores the other 70-plus neurally diverse styles of acquiring new skills, knowledge and understanding?

Dialogue as to how we can better facilitate successful learning outcomes for Autistic children cannot happen soon enough.

Children, teens and adults with Autism and an intellectual disability can and do manage to learn. It's about working to their strengths, whilst facilitating any necessary supports to aide in their learning. And as for IQ tests designed for the vast 'normal' majority…don't even get me started!

> If they can't learn the way we teach, we teach the way they learn.

O. IVAR LOVAAS

MYTH # 4 - PEOPLE ON THE SPECTRUM DON'T HAVE MEANINGFUL RELATIONSHIPS

I find the direct opposite to be true in many instances. Autistic people can make exceptionally loyal and steadfast friends. And often a shared understanding of the challenges that an Autistic experience in a 'normal' world represents, can make for unbreakable bonds within Autism families.

Those of us on The Spectrum can establish and maintain friendships that last a lifetime (particularly when we find others who share our special interests), as long as there's mutual respect for each individual's unique character.

MYTH # 5 - AUTISTIC PEOPLE DON'T WANT FRIENDS

While many of us like our own space (as all humans do on occasion!), to suggest that we all want to shut ourselves off from the world around us is of course, a misguided idea.

Our family is a perfect example of the different levels of social connection people with Autism desire. While my daughter fancies herself as a social butterfly, my son generally takes longer to warm to people – even extended family at Christmas time

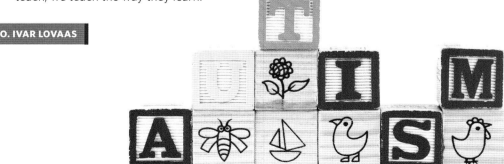

(with the exception of his beloved cousin, in which case the two are inseparable).

I prefer a happy medium, having a tendency to become mentally and emotionally fatigued by social overload. While I could never become a hermit,
I'm certainly not averse to the odd occasion of extended 'social hibernation'.

Usually these times are accompanied by periods of introspection, allowing me the necessary 'mental space' to resolve a particular problem, learn more about myself and/or move forward on my journey with renewed vigor and clarity of purpose.

MYTH # 6 - AUTISM CAN BE OUT-GROWN OR CURED

No and no. Autism is a lifelong way of being and despite all the misguided efforts of science to prove otherwise, or discover some genetic link that can be toyed with to eliminate the Autistic personality, the neuro-distinction of Autism walks among us for a reason.

MYTH # 7 - ALL AUTISTIC CHILDREN HAVE LANGUAGE DELAYS AND SPEECH ISSUES

Language delays and difficulties can be one of the common markers for Autism in infants, and some toddlers might regress in their language development at a certain age; losing speech either partially or entirely. Once again though, speech development and retention is dependent on the individual's own experience of Autism.

Our daughter had precocious language development, with a natural fascination for words that encouraged her to teach herself how to read and write stories of her own making at a very early age. Both her and our son never lost language entirely or even partially, but they do have their own communication 'quirks'.

MYTH # 8 - PEOPLE WITH AUTISM DO NOT HAVE EMPATHY

People with Autism and Asperger's are often stereotyped as insensitive 'loners', who are oblivious to the feelings of those around them.

This perception generally begins very early on, with aloof type characteristics displayed in toddlers and children often interpreted as a reluctance to engage with their family on any meaningful level.

It's also widely held that Autistic people cannot feel compassion or empathise with others. This is one of the most pervasive Autistic pathologies and in my mind, an insidious myth that's wrongly applied as a blanket trait.

One of the things we need to consider when talking to the Autistic ability or disability is how we define this very complex human experience. Empathy occurs on a number of different levels, beginning with the fundamental capacity to acknowledge that someone sees and experiences the world differently to us.

Emotional empathy occurs when we acknowledge the other person's perspective, by imagining how they feel and subsequently caring about and acknowledging their happiness, sorrow, pain and so on.

While more aloof and disconnected personality types might seem to overlook the emotional response of others and therefore not care about their feelings, I believe the opposite to be true. And I'm not alone in my beliefs.

Henry and Kamila Markram of the Swiss Federal Institute of Technology in Lausanne, claim that people on the Autism Spectrum actually feel such intense emotional responses that they must 'shut down' in order to cope.

In other words, rather than not feeling anything or very little, as has long been thought, Autistic individuals can have such an innate hypersensitivity to experiences that 'feeling overload' can overwhelm us.

Imagine walking into a room full of people and immediately being swamped with the collective energy of everyone present. This massive 'information dump' experience, is one theory behind why people with Autism seemingly avoid or disassociate from extremes of emotional exchange and social encounters. We must retreat, as it were, to process this huge volume of data.

The Markrams argue that Autistic social difficulties largely stem from trying to survive in an "intense world". Often our senses are so highly attuned that the emotional experience is magnified ten-fold.

While humming to a discontented baby might seem soothing to the 'normal' ear, for an Autistic infant this could translate to the equivalent of a heavy metal rock band performing live in their bedroom; causing a subsequent shut down of all sensory receptors.

This in turn sees the beginning of self-soothing behaviours, which generally start early in Autistic children – such as rocking, flapping and other various stims, avoiding eye contact, echoing words and actions and 'tuning out'.

Of course the problem with this reluctance to engage due to fear of sensory invasion is the potential for consistently withdrawing from interactions. This can become a pattern that takes hold, following the Autistic person throughout life and causing feelings of isolation and depression.

THE "THEORY OF MIND"

A lot of hypotheses around Autism and empathy come from what researchers call "theory of mind" - the ability to acknowledge and attribute different mental states – beliefs, desires, interests, intent, knowledge, etc – to ourselves and others. This entails recognition that not everybody thinks the same way we do, or has the same knowledge as us.

Studies suggest that people on the Spectrum develop "theory of mind" later than most non-Autistic people. Autistic children are often said to be "the centre of their own universe", particularly when it comes to talking 'at' people about their 'special interests'.

However, it isn't because we simply don't care about other people or seek to intentionally dominate the conversation, rather it's due to the perception that our interests must be universally shared.

I remember wondering if people stopped existing when I left the room, as though my presence itself animated and gave them life. This might sound a bit like a God complex, but it was a genuine concern for many years, causing me to feel overly responsible and anxious about the well-being of my entire family.

I don't think Autistic people are alone in projecting our own experiences, emotions, knowledge and thoughts on those around us. But of course for non-Autistics, presuming that everyone thinks the way you do is more likely to be an accurate assessment, given the more commonly shared neural processing.

If anything, I would argue that Autism presents as an empathy overload.

When teachers yelled at other children in the classroom, I felt as though I had been personally reprimanded. And anything remotely 'hurtful' that's said or done to me is internalised and anguished over for months (sometimes years).

To this day I will never, no matter how curious I might be, enquire as to the price someone paid for anything I might find particularly interesting. I have a vivid memory of my sister reprimanding me for doing so at about the age of twelve, when I innocently asked our cousin how much the new leather jacket she was sporting (and I was admiring) had cost.

At the time, the shame I felt was devastating. But I still have no idea why my asking this question had upset my sister so much, or why it's apparently considered poor social etiquette.

I've been taken advantage of more times than I care to admit, wrongly assuming that everyone is like me, failing to recognise and understand self-serving agendas. My experiences of betrayal and bullying have left indelible scars, because these acts cut deep to the sensitive soul.

IN CONCLUSION

No two Autistic experiences of the world are ever alike. We need to look less to pathologised definitions of "Autism" and more to the experience of Autistic individuals in order to guide the facilitation of their most capable and full life.

You're all geniuses, and you're all beautiful. You don't need anyone to tell you who you are. You are what you are. Get out there and get peace, think peace, and live peace and breathe peace, and you'll get it as soon as you like.

JOHN LENNON

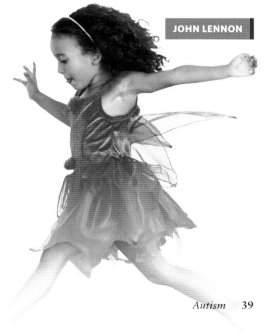

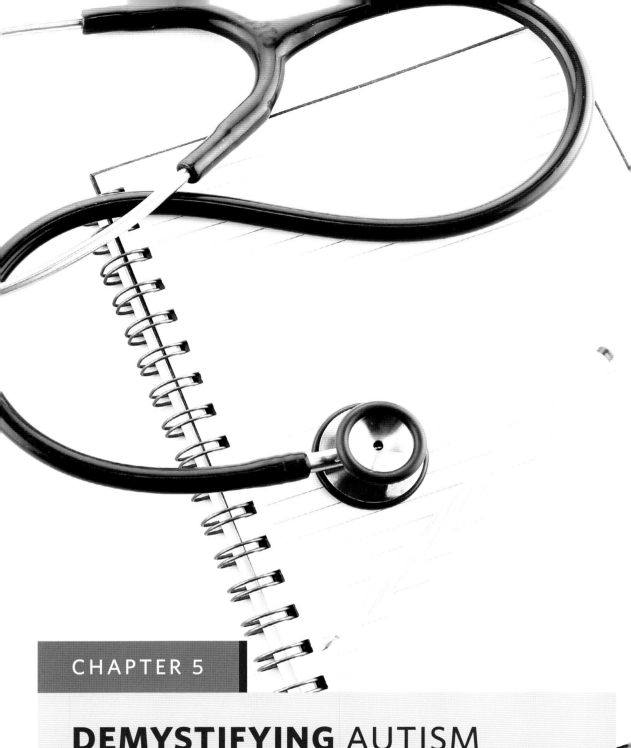

CHAPTER 5

DEMYSTIFYING AUTISM
ASSESSMENT AND DIAGNOSIS

Diagnosis, for our family, was a double-edged sword. In one way it was a blessing – we were vindicated in our arguments with numerous medical professionals whose initial assessment of Aislinn was simply silent reflux.

On the other hand, we had unwittingly bestowed upon her a label that's all too often (unjustly) synonymous with lifelong limitations.

Over the last decade or so, Autism diagnostic rates have been on a steadily rapid incline across the world. Reasons for the apparent escalation are varied and based largely on conjecture. Some of the more popular theories include:

- Better awareness and understanding of what Autism is and therefore less chance of some other 'disorder' or 'mental illness' being wrongly diagnosed.
- More knowledgeable medical professionals who are better able to identify early 'signs', including Maternal and Child Health staff.
- Environmental and/or genetic influences creating a rise in the incidents of Autism.

Whatever the reasons, the numbers seem to indicate that the rate of diagnosis in children across many developed countries has increased by about 30% over the past five or so years.

SHOULD I SEEK AN ASSESSMENT?

Initial signs of Autism can often mirror other developmental differences, including things like hearing issues. However there are a number of recognised 'red flag' characteristics in the Autistic toddler that are absent in children who exhibit, say, delayed speech in isolation.

Most of these more unique markers are around social interaction. But the journey is different for everybody. For us, the first signs were largely to do with sleep and sensory issues.

As a baby Aislinn could scream for hours on end. She often seemed inconsolable and appeared to experience extreme discomfort when nursing. She remained awake and alert for long stretches, often cat napping in our arms, but waking as soon as we attempted to lay her down.

She hated the car and walks in the pusher, confounding many armchair experts who insisted both modes of travel would prove soothing for any baby. She also had a penchant for eighties glam rock (think Poison and Bon Jovi), rather than classical music or nursery rhymes.

Despite no consistent, notable indicators of silent reflux, the paediatrician we initially approached (desperate for help) insisted she should be medicated. When, at about 5 months of age, the medication had made no discernible difference, they did an invasive barium swallow. This yielded a result that suggested no obvious signs of reflux or regurgitation whatsoever.

Rather than admit defeat, our paediatrician consulted his colleague who, just as perplexed by Aislinn's presentation, informed me that I was perhaps a 'beef cow' rather than a 'dairy cow' and prescribed specialist formula.

All of this to-ing and fro-ing saw our daughter's extremes of sleep and sensory disturbances continue for the next two years, without any real answers.

Often parents will start noticing differences with their children quite early on and even from birth (as was the case with us). Regularly scheduled visits with a MCHN or family doctor, to routinely monitor 'normal' infant development, can trigger questions if certain milestones seem to go unmet.

Aislinn's first indicators were fussiness around feeding, fairly regular bouts of distress, demonstrated by incredibly loud screaming for anything up to nine hours straight, constant sleep issues and severe separation anxiety.

Then there was the debilitating fear of loud noises and seeming reluctance to acknowledge or interact with other children in the mum's group we attended. Aislinn's language development was atypical in that she could speak in four word sentences by around 22 months of age.

We had to (and still do) repeat her name multiple times before gaining her attention, and she can often seem oblivious to our attempts at establishing lines of communication. Then just when you think she's not paying any heed, she'll mention something said in passing three weeks ago!

Interestingly (and very tellingly), my brother was the first 'outside observer' to voice what we had long suspected when he watched Aislinn, at the age of about fourteen months, race across the lawn on her tip toes. When she remained on the balls of her feet for the entire duration of his visit, he very matter-of-factly declared – "Yep, Asperger's right there."

Different researchers are studying further Autistic 'tells', such as distinct anomalies in gait, observed when the child walks and runs.

Does age matter?

The average age of diagnosis in the United States is currently 4 years, however recent studies suggest the 'telltale signs' of Autism can be observed in children as young as 2.

This is causing medical specialists involved in Autism assessment to re-evaluate the long-held belief that diagnosis should be delayed until the child is closer to school age, when they're consistently exposed to social encounters that could highlight signs of the Autistic pathology.

Emphasis is increasingly centred on earlier diagnosis, with studies exploring how babies under twelve months can possibly be accurately assessed using different observational methods.

This turnaround is due to extensive research, which suggests that the earlier 'interventions' are applied to Autistic children; the more potential there is for better life outcomes in the long run.

Of course this means different things to different people. But you already know what it means to me, in the context of this book.

SIGNS YOUR CHILD MIGHT BE ON THE SPECTRUM OF DIFFERENCE

Following are some of the more 'common signs' acknowledged as early indicators of Autism. Given that, as I have mentioned previously, Autism is a spectrum – a continuum of different experiences and different extremes of those experiences – not every child will display every characteristic.

- Seems non-responsive & doesn't display affection to caregivers in usual ways – i.e. Doesn't indicate desire to be picked up, lack of eye contact, doesn't outwardly express emotion and seems to shy away from touch.
- Lack of interest in other children, doesn't smile at others, 'ignores' or appears indifferent to people around them, doesn't develop 'normal' peer relations and is reluctant to join in activities.
- Seems to be in 'own world' and can have extremes of behaviours, along with anxiety type experiences.
- Variables in verbal communication, including delayed or no speech, patterns of 'normal' speech followed by loss of some or all acquired words, echolalia (mimicking) and literal interpretation.

On the flipside, verbal language development may appear precocious or advanced, with an apparent accompanying lack of comprehension as to the meaning and messages conveyed by the range of words used – i.e. verbal scope does not match scope of comprehension somehow. This was very much the case with Aislinn. Other indicators can include:

- Unusual and repetitive attachments to objects or topics – some examples in our household include trains, Lego, loom bands, drawing (and within the drawings themselves, repetitive preoccupations with different subjects).
- Hyper or hypo-sensitivity to noise and pain.
- Food fads and fussiness.
- Sleep disturbances and difficulty settling.
- Unusual fears and in particular, fear of loud noises such as vacuum cleaners and lawn mowers.
- Mouthing of objects, beyond the commonly accepted age for 'normal' development in this area.
- Seems distant and quiet – this one aligns with an apparent "lack of curiosity". In my experience, the curious Autistic mind is highly attuned for observation, hence we can become "distant and quiet" when processing all that's observed in minute detail.
- May have a tendency to wander – my brother was known for "losing mum" at least once during every shopping outing as a child.
- May seek or avoid body contact and "rough and tumble" play.
- May appear clumsy and uncoordinated.
- Muscle tone may appear 'poor' or 'weak'.
- Could have what appears to be 'obsessive' behaviours and interests, including playing with toys in unusual ways – e.g. Only spinning tyres on toy cars, lining up blocks in colour sequences, etc.

EARLY INDICATORS

Numerous studies are emerging to suggest that Autism can be identified in children as young as 2 years of age, when it's believed they start exhibiting a number of distinct differences around movement, communication, emotional control and problem solving.

In one study (Feb 2014 Rosa Milagros Santos et al, University of Illinois – Early Childhood Longitudinal Study, Birth Cohort), researchers examined around 100 children with Autism, a further 1,100 with disabilities like hearing impairments or intellectual disability and 7,700 "typically developing" children.

They found that at 9 months of age, children later diagnosed with Autism were more likely than their non-Autistic counterparts to wake three or more times during the night.

At two years of age, the same children were more likely to transition quickly from whimpering to full-blown crying (leading researchers to hypothesise difficulty managing emotions), and less words were being used – 10, compared with about 22 for children with a disability and 30 for the control subjects.

Other distinctions in two year old children who went on to receive an Autism diagnosis included;

- Difficulty naming objects, listening to others and recognising and using words.
- Not as proficient at matching colours or using numbers as those in other groups (although our daughter and other children I know have grown up to become quite the little mathematicians!).
- Apparent motor coordination delays, including floppy arms, difficulty sitting up and grasping and manipulating small objects.
- Smiling less and crying more when interacting with their mothers.
- More inclined to continue playing with one toy rather than reaching for others.
- More easily frustrated and less persistent and cooperative than children in the two other groups.
- Showed more signs of requiring constant attention and experiencing separation anxiety.

NAVIGATING THE AUTISM ASSESSMENT JOURNEY

Autism is generally diagnosed by comparing certain developmental and behavioural characteristics with pathologised symptoms, as outlined in the Diagnostic and Statistical Manual (DSM) of the day (although some countries have variations in criteria).

In May 2013, a revised DSM-5 introduced significant changes to Autism assessment protocol, including the removal of Asperger Syndrome and Pervasive Developmental Disorder – Not Otherwise Specified (PDD-NOS) from the recognised Autism Spectrum.

Now to qualify for a diagnosis, parents or the patient (if an adult is being retrospectively diagnosed) must report persistent deficits (note negative pathologised language) in social communication and interaction across a range of contexts, which could not be attributed to some other type of developmental delay.

This is essentially a process of 'ticking' the following boxes:

- Nonverbal communication issues – abnormal eye contact, posture, facial expressions, tone of voice and gestures, as well as a seeming inability to understand how and why they are used when engaging with others.
- Social interaction issues - Problems reciprocating social or emotional interaction, including;
    - Difficulty establishing or maintaining back-and-forth conversations
    - Inability to initiate interactions with others
    - Problems sharing interests and emotions with others
- Problems maintaining relationships - Including lack of interest in others and difficulties around the areas of pretend play, engaging in age-appropriate social activities and adjusting to various social expectations.

There must also be two of the following four characteristics related to restricted and repetitive behaviour present for an Autism diagnosis:

- Repetitive or stereotyped speech, use of objects or motor movement.
- Strict and excessive adherence to routines, ritualised patterns of nonverbal and/or verbal behaviour, or complete resistance to change.
- Highly restricted interests, abnormal in intensity and focus.
- Hyper or hypo sensitivity, demonstrated by extreme reactions to different sensory input and stimuli and/or an unusual interest in sensory aspects of the environment.

FURTHER CHANGES TO DIAGNOSIS

The DSM-5 introduced a few further annotations around the pathology of Autism and how it's assessed and ultimately diagnosed, including:

1. Recognised co-morbidities

Unlike its predecessor, the new diagnostic manual allows for two or more 'disorders' to be diagnosed as 'co-morbidities' that sit side by side, such as ASD and ADHD.

2. New diagnosis of Social Communication Disorder (SCD)

Under the old DSM-4, a child who presented with developmental delays around social communication, but who didn't quite meet the other ASD criteria, were either given the label of PDD-NOS or went undiagnosed.

The DSM-5 presents the new option of SCD, with the main distinction between ASD and SCD being that the child diagnosed with SCD doesn't demonstrate persistent, repetitive behaviours.

3. Effects of symptoms

The symptoms, while possibly not becoming fully apparent until social demand exceeds capacity (eg. Schooling begins), must be present in early childhood, functionally impairing and not better described by a different diagnosis.

4. Severity scale applied

Symptoms are given a severity ranking, whereby 1 is severe and 3 is mild, according to the perceived impact on a person's ability to 'function normally' and how debilitating the impairment is considered.

The ranking is determined by the level of expected support the patient might need, now and in the future. While many hope this will see the application of more appropriately targeted 'treatments' and 'interventions' for Autistic individuals, simplifying everyone down to a one to three numbered ranking still doesn't cut the mustard in my book. Or should I say, the "fruit salad"?

The DSM's ranking also reflects the impact of any co-morbidities or co-occurring diagnoses, such as intellectual disabilities, language impairment and medical and other behavioural challenges.

There is no single test available to effectively diagnose Autism. Assessment is based on:

1. Observing how the child interacts and plays with others – this may be done in a professional or home environment.
2. Reviewing their developmental history and looking for any notable differences in achieving recognised milestones.
3. Parent/carer interviews and testimonial to provide insight into behaviours and interactions with significant caregivers at home.

Clinicians use different locally and internationally recognised screening and measurement tools to test for Autistic traits and arrive at a diagnosis, depending on the country you live in, such as:

- Childhood Autism Rating Scales (CARS)
- Autism Behaviour Checklist (ABC)
- Autism Diagnostic Interview (ADI)
- Autism Diagnostic Observation Schedule (ADOS)
- Developmental Behaviour Checklist (DBC)
- Modified Checklist for Autism in Toddlers (M-CHAT)
- Psycho-Educational Profile – Revised (PEP-R)
- Social Communication Questionnaire (SCQ)

The assessment and subsequent diagnosis of ASD can be a long and arduous journey, so we look at how to successfully navigate each step and what to do beyond a diagnosis in the following chapter. For now, let's break it down into digestible pieces that will hopefully make it less daunting.

STEP BY STEP ASSESSMENT GUIDE

Following is an outline to help you navigate the various medical processes and professionals you are likely to encounter at some stage during your Autism assessment journey.

Because criteria, testing tools and diagnostic protocols differ across the world, there may be some localised variations to this roadmap for you and your child. For specific information based on where you live, please contact your local Autism support network or official peak body.

In the beginning

Chances are the first conversation you have about Autism and your child will be with your maternal health nurse, a pre-school teacher, childcare worker, or a primary school teacher.

Usually parents notice signs that their child is 'different', however it may take prompting from a trusted person outside of the immediate family to set the assessment wheels in motion.

The first step is a visit to your family doctor to obtain a referral to an appropriate specialist or team of multi-disciplinary specialists.

Generally diagnosis will not be readily considered prior to the child turning 2 years, with average age of diagnosis occurring at around the 4-year mark.

Who is involved?

For a clinical diagnosis to be officially recognised, it must come from a paediatrician, psychologist and/or psychiatrist. They will observe your child and speak to you at length about their developmental and behavioural history in order to uncover any potential Autistic traits and patterns.

Multidisciplinary assessment

Given that Autism assessment relies on more than ticking a few medical boxes, the specialist you see is likely to refer you on to professionals in other fields of practice for various screening tests.

Depending on which country you reside in, children and their parents may be eligible to access government funding for so-called 'early interventions'. In some instances, to qualify for such financial assistance a multi-disciplinary diagnosis is essential.

A multi-disciplinary assessment team usually involves one of the above specialists as well as:

An Occupational Therapist (OT) – trained health professionals who work with Autistic 'patients' to assess and address any developmental delays that may impede daily activities, such as eating, dressing, toileting, managing personal hygiene, partaking in activities and schooling.

OT's can also complete a comprehensive sensory profile for your child to indicate their sensory seeking and avoiding patterns. They can then work through these and teach you and your child how to effectively manage sensory induced anxiety and behaviours.

The word "Autistic" is accurate. But so are other words that we no longer use to describe people: spinster (unmarried woman), hobo (migrant worker), cripple (person with a physical handicap), and so on. The fact that a person is unmarried or has sustained a mobility-reducing injury or birth defect certainly figures into their life experiences, but it does not define their character—unless they or we let it.

ELLEN NOTBOHM

A Speech Therapist or Speech Pathologist – Whether a child is verbal or non-verbal, they will usually see a trained speech pathologist to undertake a language assessment.

Speech therapists use various tests to ascertain a child's developmental ability with regard to the recognised 'norms' of verbal and non-verbal communication, as well as things like pragmatic language comprehension.

Cognitive Assessment in Autism

I'm not a fan of standardised IQ testing, as it fails to account for innate Autistic differences in processing the world, and potential barriers due to language and behavioural interference.

I've heard of numerous instances where a child has scored below 70 at a young age, only to develop into a mathematical or technical genius a few years later.

However, IQ tests are often used to indicate whether the child might have an intellectual disability as well as Autism, along with their cognitive strengths and weaknesses.

In Australia, how a child scores on his or her IQ test will determine whether they have access to a funded aide in the classroom during their primary and secondary schooling, so cognitive assessment is usually done at time of diagnosis or soon after.

Studies have shown that about half of people with Autism score below 50 on IQ tests, while 20% score between 50 and 70 and 30% score above 70, with a small percentage scoring in the gifted range (around the 98 or above percentile). I take all of these statistics with a grain of salt.

Financial considerations and timing

One of the most controversial areas of Autism assessment and diagnosis across many developed countries, is the financial burden that families often face when undertaking complex and time consuming intensive assessment, diagnostic and therapy regimes.

In Australia, as is also the case in places like Canada and the UK, parents have the choice of a private or public healthcare assessment. While the former option potentially costs thousands of dollars, but represents a hastier diagnostic pathway, the latter can be a cheaper but lengthier alternative.

If you decide to use the public system, chances are you will be put on waiting lists to access the necessary specialists, with assessment sometimes taking up to a year or more.

As such, it's worthwhile to start making appointments as soon as possible, irrespective of whether you have all of your referral letters organised or not.

On the flipside, if you feel a diagnosis is time critical – as is often the case with parents seeking answers for their children who might be struggling at a pivotal social point, like transitioning to school – privately accessed practitioners will provide a quicker outcome, but can cost anywhere up to $2000 to $5000 per child.

Australia's current public health system provides parents with various options for financial assistance in navigating the assessment process, partially covering the associated specialist costs in some instances. So it's worth doing some research and speaking at length to your GP (General Practitioner) about this.

THE FUTURE OF AUTISM ASSESSMENT

Many professionals believe that one of the fundamental flaws with current Autism assessment protocols is the reliance on parent observation, as well as how treating practitioners translate parent testimonial into a comprehensive diagnosis.

Frequently there are different interpretations of criteria applied, depending on the specialist consulted, causing many to suggest that the process in its current form is flawed and unreliable.

Researchers continue working toward alternative, biological means of assessing Autism, including the possibility of detecting Autistic markers through blood tests to measure protein levels and gauge an individuals' 'protein fingerprint', which studies have shown to be consistently and markedly different in people with Autism.

This type of screening is still far from becoming widely available to clinicians, and many question the moral and ethical implications of such tests if applied (as a lot of scientific and genetic research is working toward) to prenatal testing in a bid to determine a child's likelihood of developing Autistic traits.

Our community must engage in serious and meaningful dialogue as to the need for us to continue pathologising and subsequently diagnosing and labelling what is actually a neurologically diverse social minority.

I find it difficult to conceptualise living in a world that insists people's needs cannot be met or their disability experience of this world recognised and acknowledged on any truly empathic, individual basis, unless they are said to be "suffering" from Autism as some type of disease.

Think of it: a disability is usually defined in terms of what is missing... But Autism... is as much about what is abundant as what is missing, an over-expression of the very traits that make our species unique.

PAUL COLLINS

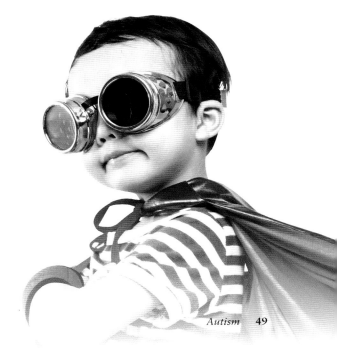

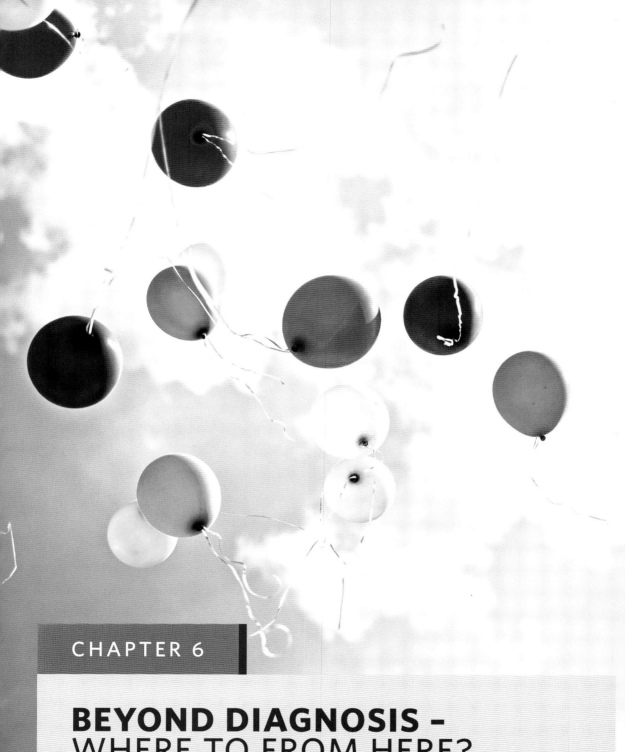

CHAPTER 6

BEYOND DIAGNOSIS –
WHERE TO FROM HERE?

For many parents, receiving an official Autism diagnosis for their child can be confronting. Feelings of grief, loss, anger and guilt can intermingle with confusion about where to go and what to do from this point on.

Some have compared the experience to a type of mourning, whereby parents are forced to let go of the preconceived ideas and expectations they had been harbouring about their children's future(s) and what their family would look like.

While I understand this very emotional response, I would suggest that having to put away those expectations of your child is actually a very positive, empowering thing to do. Because it means allowing them to define who they are and determine their own path through this world. And remember, while that path may not look like everyone else's, it's just as worthy.

An Autism diagnosis might be the end of the world – as you know it – but it's also the beginning of a whole new journey. Your life will never be the same again. There will be ups and downs, laughter and tears, happiness and sorrow…but it will all be worthwhile and make you a better person if you let it.

An Autism diagnosis can be acknowledged as a time of regrets and grief, or a time of reflection and growth. We cannot choose whether Autism is a part of our lives, but we can choose how we travel this path as parents. And that will make all the difference.

1. DEALING WITH A DIAGNOSIS

When speaking with parents who are battling mixed feelings about a diagnosis, I ask them to acknowledge that this is still the same little boy or girl they have loved unconditionally since they were born. The word 'Autism' does not change who they are, or the meaning they have in your world.

Much of the sadness and uncertainty that surrounds a diagnosis is due to that pervasive Autistic stereotype, and the oftentimes-negative prognosis provided by medical professionals. Usually you will hear 'worse case scenarios' or, just as potentially undermining to the child's life experience, stories of Autistic savants and giftedness.

What ensues is the placement of expectations on your child that can fundamentally change and restrict how you interact with them and in turn, how they develop throughout their most formative years.

Suddenly precious little Isabel or Jack isn't a person with his or her own defining character anymore. They are reduced to a word – they are 'Autistic'. Try applying a label to an object and not defining its purpose based on the label itself.

We call a cup a cup and define its purpose as holding liquid beverages. But if you were to serve someone cheese and crackers from a cup, they would be perplexed by your unusual application of what we recognise as a drinking vessel. Their brain, conditioned over time, has an expectation of 'normal' use for said cup and anything that deviates from that expectation challenges our lifelong conditioning.

This is the same for 'Autism', which is identified by a list of things the Autistic person is incapable of or 'deficient' in. By doing so, we underestimate their potential, denying them the right and opportunity to discover who they really are and their life's purpose.

Comparing Autistic children with their non-Autistic peers or even another Autistic child, in terms of their capabilities and personalities, is like comparing apples and oranges. It's an injustice for, not only the child and you as their parent, but also the world and everyone else in it.

When we deny our own natural growth and evolution as individuals, we potentially deny the evolution of our entire planet. Who knows what difference your child's own unique difference could make in this lifetime? Who knows what impact they could have on this world and those around them?

> What would happen if the Autism gene was eliminated from the gene pool? You would have a bunch of people standing around in a cave, chatting and socializing and not getting anything done.

TEMPLE GRANDIN

It isn't up to us to tell them what they are, it's up to us, as parents, to nurture these little souls and encourage them to discover who they are for themselves. That's the role of every parent.

Remember, a diagnosis doesn't define your child and shouldn't be used as a comparative yardstick against other 'normally developing' children.

If you are compelled to seek a diagnosis, use it to empower yourself and your child. In understanding your child's difference, you can equip them with the necessary tools and learning to facilitate their most successful life possible – whatever that might look like.

With that in mind, here are my four top tips to make an Autism diagnosis a journey of personal growth, rather than a process of grieving:

1. Be encouraged and empowered. This isn't the end of your child's world or journey in life…It's simply a different beginning.

2. Formulate an action plan that will encourage your child's development into the person they have the potential to become. This might include different play-based activities or therapies guided by specialists. But remember, each child is individual and will have different needs based on his or her own unique "fruit salad", so don't settle for a 'one size fits all' approach – more on this later.

3. Rally the troops! You will need support from family and friends at this time, but avoid falling into negative, no-end discussions about the diagnosis and your child's pathology. Focus on them as a little person and stay positive, educating those around you and your child as to the potentials and possibilities of the

Autistic experience, rather than a list of 'problems'.

Build a trusted network of support around your child – people who will encourage them to believe they are capable and valued, talking to their strengths and helping them work on those areas where they need assistance.

4. Do some homework. There is no shortage of books and blogs on the Internet, as well as great social networking groups and forums that can provide first hand insight into life on the Autism Spectrum.

    Balance your reading of books and information on the Internet from academics and medical professionals with inspiring, real life recollections and stories from the true experts on Autism – Autistic people and their supportive families.

Finally, it's important to remember that a diagnosis isn't a reflection on you as a parent. Don't get bogged down in a cycle of questioning why this has happened to your family, or looking for something or someone to blame. Instead, focus on what you can do in the here and now and take each day as it comes. Autism is a great reminder that life is about living in the moment.

2. WHAT DOES A DIAGNOSIS MEAN FOR YOU AND YOUR FAMILY OR CHILD?

The most common question I receive from parents who have a newly diagnosed child is, "What now?"

All too often, a report is received confirming your child has Autism, without any clear direction as to where you can go to seek out necessary supports.

As such, parents are left with little option but to try to figure it all out for themselves, which often means trawling through information found on Google that can perpetuate these disheartening prognoses for your family's future.

Statistics trotted out by high profile, peak bodies in various countries inform us that:

* The cost of providing care for a person with Autism is an estimated US$3.2 million over their lifetime. The cost of Autism per year for families is approximately $60,000.
* Families with Autistic children are likely to earn 28% less overall compared with 'normal' families, as often one or both parents will have to sacrifice full time work for full time care of their child.
* 66% of adults on the Autism Spectrum remain unemployed.
* Only around 56% of children with Autism will successfully complete schooling and graduate from higher education.
* Only 17% of young adults with Autism (between 21 and 25 years of age) have ever lived on their own, compared with 66% who had learning disabilities like dyslexia.
* 80% of marriages, where one or more children in the family have Autism, end in divorce.

What I find interesting about these types of studies is that they usually rely on restricted sets of data around small subgroups from within the Autism community. However, the media reports them with great authority, as reliable evidence to continue perpetuating negative Autistic stereotypes.

I won't deny that there are real and often exhausting challenges when it comes to living with Autism – for the Autistic person as well as their loved ones.

But let's face it, every family has obstacles to overcome and the fact remains that raising children is an expensive and exhausting learning curve, Autism or no. It's also the greatest blessing and privilege we can experience in life.

Some of these research findings are now being openly questioned for their accuracy and reliability, as well as the detrimental effects such negative "promotion" of Autism is having on millions of families around the world.

In 2010, the Centre for Autism and Related Disorders at the Kennedy Krieger Institute in Baltimore (US) debunked the myth that parents of a child with Autism were more likely to separate, with 80% of marriages ending in divorce.

Their research found that children with Autism remained with either both biological or adoptive parents 64% of the time, not unlike non-Autistic families where children remain with both parents (biological or adoptive) 65% of the time.

While Autism has the potential to strengthen families who resolve to work together and support one another throughout their own unique journey, it cannot and should not be held accountable for destroying relationships.

Autistic children, teens and adults have been 'easy targets' to blame for numerous social issues for far too long. It's time we started to turn this cause and effect argument on its head; acknowledging that many of the social expectations surrounding today's perceptions of 'normal' human behaviour, actually perpetuate Autistic stigmas and create barriers to meaningful neuro-atypical experience in a world of 'sameness'.

SIBLING SURVIVAL TIPS

One of the most difficult things to juggle in a family where one or more children have Autism can be the 'fair and equitable' division of attention.

I know from personal experience that our daughter, who is far more prone to daily bouts of anxiety due to sensory and other triggers, can consume hours of our time. Likewise, her and her younger brother's sleep disturbances that wake us in the middle of the night can leave us fatigued and incapable of basic human function on some occasions!

I've had many guilt addled moments thinking that we've neglected our two boys, who are less emotionally demonstrative and can therefore be overlooked from time to time, as we help Aislinn better understand and manage her feelings and sensory triggers.

As a parent you want your children to love one another and be close. So how do you foster healthy sibling relationships in Spectrum families? Here are my five tips to maintain healthy sibling relationships:

1. Make time – it's easy to become consumed with all the 'things' on our 'To do' lists. And if you have a child undergoing some type of therapy, your 'To do' list can seem exhausting and endless. It's important to take some time out just to be with your children in the moment – whether it's reading a book, playing their favourite game or watching a movie.

You might allocate special time for each child. Just make these goals realistic and achievable, because creating unrealistic expectations will only lead to further feelings of anguish and guilt (been there, done that!).

2. Be kind to you – no one likes a grumpy mum or dad. It can be difficult to manage daily emotions and stresses when you neglect your own needs constantly.

However I'm not going to preach to you about having some 'me time'. Why? Because I know for some parents, it can be nigh on impossible to even finish a cup of tea before it goes cold, or go to the bathroom without an audience in tow!

Taking time out to recharge can be tricky for any parent, let alone those of us who assume the role of full time carer and/ or teacher for our children. But if you find the right

support network and resources in your community, you should be able to achieve some type of well-deserved break.

Even if it means taking half an hour to read a book or meditate when everyone else has gone to bed, just be kind to you and remind yourself that you are doing the best possible job you can. We tend to focus more on our perceived 'mistakes', but it's essential that you acknowledge your family's accomplishments and growth as you journey a little further every day.

By all means learn from your mistakes, but don't beat yourself up over them!

3. Encourage their interests – one of the dangers with Autism is how all-consuming it can become. Avoid everyone's lives being defined by Autism and the perceived impositions it brings by nurturing the interests of other children in your family. This also gives siblings of Autistic children an outlet, where they can establish other relationships and start to build their own identity.

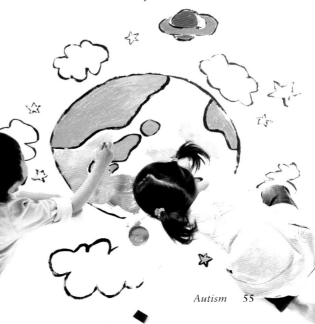

4. Don't make Autism the family burden to bear – this is so important! It's easy to slip into a cycle where you perpetuate the negative perceptions of Autism with your own beliefs and attitudes.

Avoid defining your family's experience by the many talked about restrictions of Autism. Focus instead on your strengths and the solutions and accomplishments you are all capable of achieving when working together, as a cohesive, loving and cooperative family unit.

You will be doing your children a great service by instilling this lesson of collaborative problem sharing and solving from a young age.

Finding the balance in your household will take practice and a good deal of trial and error. But it's a worthwhile balance to strike. While it's not advisable to delegate too many care responsibilities to siblings, who could start to resent their brother or sister and treat them differently, instilling the virtues of patience, empathy and understanding by openly talking with them about their own experience of Autism will make them more compassionate human beings in the long run. Something the world definitely needs more of!

3. HOW TO AVOID THE "BLAME AND SHAME GAME"

Although the 'cause' of Autism remains elusive, academics and researchers have tabled numerous theories over time and continue to seek 'the answer'.

From older dads, to exposure to labour inducing hormones in utero and environmental toxins, expert conjecture abounds as to why some children are born Autistic. One thing the experts agree on is that genetics plays a very important part; to what degree and how exactly is still up for debate however.

More often than not, searching for a clear answer as to what 'caused' your child's Autism will result in a process of attributing blame to one another as parents.

This is an all too common scenario I see and hear played out. Fathers or mothers believe they have 'given' their child Autism and either refuse to acknowledge the diagnosis, or start to resent one another for contributing to the perceived 'problems' their child has.

When you add different cultural perceptions to the mix, where 'disability' might be viewed as a blight on the family name, the blaming and shaming can be enough to cripple relationships.

Rather than seeking answers as to why Autism is a part of your lives, this is a time when parents need to resolve and be strong in their commitment to working together, so that you may help your child grow into the person they are capable of becoming.

Maintain and grow your relationship as a couple by pro-actively reinforcing the bonds that brought you together in the first instance and;

1. Acknowledge and talk about how Autism looks in your household and what it means for everyone. Remember

you are not alone on this journey, so seek out networks of other parents in your community who understand and support you – this is important for both mums and dads, with the latter often being overlooked in their carer role and needs.

2. Talk about other stuff! One of the most difficult things in an Autism household is avoiding the potential for Autism to completely consume your every waking moment. Remember that you are both your own persons with your own unique character and interests. Maintain your respective identities by revisiting those qualities that attracted you to one another before children entered your world.

3. Maintain a united front. Keep your relationship strong by communicating your feelings with one another every day and talking through any problems you encounter as a team.

4. Focus on solutions. Avoid getting bogged down in 'problem talk' by persisting to find solutions instead. Talk through challenging situations and use one another's identified strengths to overcome them.

5. Take time to be a couple. We don't all have the means to get dressed up and go on a regular 'date night' - this is true. But even if it's just spending half an hour in quiet conversation, a small show of affection as you pass one another in the hallway, or watching a movie in quiet contemplation, it's critical to maintain your own connection and make your relationship a priority whenever you can.

6. Acknowledge and encourage one another. All too often we take our loved ones for granted. Take some time to reflect on how far you have come on your journey as a family and how you have all contributed to that remarkable growth.

4. TAKING POSITIVE ACTION AND AVOIDING "DIAGNOSIS DEPRESSION"

While it's necessary and healthy to acknowledge any feelings you might experience as the result of your child's Autism diagnosis, diving into a pit of despair is never ideal.

Should you sense yourself slipping into bouts of moodiness or tearing up for no apparent reason on a regular basis, it might be time to seek help of some kind.

In most countries, you will be able to access family counsellors and therapists via your local Autism organisation or support network, so this can be a great place to start when looking for someone to talk to.

Taking positive action and empowering yourself with information will go a long way to staving off feelings of helplessness, and seeking out support from others who are living the Autism journey is a good way to avoid social isolation.

Most importantly, now is the time to contemplate your first 'next steps' after diagnosis and from there, establish a clear plan of action to maintain forward momentum with an assertive, confident and positive attitude – the most important weapon in your arsenal as carer and advocate for your child!

5. THE FIRST "NEXT STEPS"

In no particular order…

1. **Take some time to digest and reflect** on your child's diagnosis before you dive headlong into an 'intervention' or 'therapy' plan. Based on the report you get outlining the areas where they might have difficulties, do some research into what could potentially benefit your child in addressing their challenges and building on their attributes.

2. It might sound a little strange, but it can help to sit down and **create a "personality profile" for your child** – list those attributes that make them loveable, along with any Autistic traits that could prove challenging for them in this world. There will be many occasions where you are asked to focus on the perceived 'deficiencies' of your child's Autism. It's important to have this information at hand, but even more important to balance out the 'bad' with a healthy dose of the 'good'.

3. **Understand your child's sensory profile and behavioural triggers.** Autistic children are not willfully defiant or naughty, as is often mistakenly believed. Rather, their behaviours are a direct reflection of their experiences in this world and in particular the various sensory triggers they are constantly exposed to.

   By understanding what environmental triggers might cause a 'meltdown', you can better equip yourself to manage destructive or harmful behaviours and are less likely to react by trying to discipline your child in these moments, which will be ineffective at best and escalate undesirable behaviours at worst.

4. **Find out what funding you might be entitled to.** Depending on the country in which you reside and the age of your child, he or she might qualify for financial assistance to access interventions and therapies. You could also be entitled to carer payments or subsidies from the government.

5. **Consider a treatment plan.** Generally when families receive a diagnosis they will be informed of a few therapeutic approaches to support their child's social, emotional and psychological development, as well as his or her capacity for learning and assimilating with peers.

   However, numerous 'non-evidence-based' approaches are proving very effective for many families nowadays. While these are not necessarily recognised as 'conventional' practices, some parents feel that more empathetic 'interventions' better align with nurturing their child's diversity constructively.

   Irrespective of the course you decide to pursue, it's critical that you do your homework, understand what is involved in terms of time, resources and costs and importantly, make sure the treatment isn't going to endanger your child's physical, mental or emotional wellbeing in any way. And please don't buy into expensive treatment regimes in response to the Autism stigma!

> If we can't see a child with Autism as capable, interesting and valuable, no amount of therapy we layer on top is going to matter.

ELLEN NOTBOHM

6. **Be proactive rather than reactive.** One of the most difficult things to overcome, as the parent of an Autistic child, is the belief that behavioural issues can be disciplined in the same way a 'tantrum' might be.

   We had to throw out the rulebook and approach things very differently to how our parents raised us when it came to managing Aislinn's behaviours – the ones her anxiety and sensory issues trigger.

   Children on the Spectrum can still have standard "I want" tantrums too, so the idea is to learn how to distinguish them. This is about observing and understanding the underlying 'language' of behaviours, which are essentially another form of communication.

   Children on the Spectrum generally thrive on boundaries and routine and I personally find that a direct, no-nonsense approach that speaks to their logical mind is the most well received when it comes to guiding them safely through life.

   Set clear routines and boundaries that your children can learn to rely on, which will in turn make them feel more secure. Try to find ways to address behaviours before they escalate and seek out help to do so wherever necessary. If you can maintain a proactive approach, you are less likely to become reactionary and in turn, overwhelmed by certain behaviours.

7. **Broaden your support network.** Seek out Autism specific support groups in your local neighbourhood if possible, or if you are geographically isolated, find a Facebook group or Internet forum where you can 'talk' with other parents who understand the Autism journey, as well as Autistic adults and mentors. I have seen many wonderful friendships flourish within these types of environments and the encouragement and understanding you find among the Autism community is invaluable.

8. **Avoid paralysis by analysis** – become a critical, thinking consumer of information and avoid getting bogged down in all the literature that abounds on Autism. Sift through and focus on relevant resources specific to your experience, or insights that give you a "light bulb" moment. Be selective in what you do with advice, whether offered or uncovered in your research.

   Most of all don't stop moving forward on your journey due to information overload, or fear of what to do with the knowledge you acquire. If you get stuck on something, the best thing to do is seek out someone from your support network to discuss it with, whether it's a new therapy you're considering or some type of day to day concern.

9. **Resolve to become your child's champion.** One of the first things Aislinn's occupational therapist said to me was that I would be her lifelong advocate. It was and is up to us as parents, to ensure our children have fair and equitable access to the same resources and opportunities as every other child.

    Understand your rights and the rights of your child in various social settings and systems and have a clear knowledge of their specific needs, so that you can inform others appropriately.

    I smile every day watching my own kids grow and blossom, and the more they progress, the stronger an advocate I become for those who don't have a voice.

    MATT BENTGZEN,
    father of two sons with Asperger's

10. **Seek out supports for your child within the local community.** If they are not yet school age, contact your local early intervention worker and find out what type of services they offer that might be of benefit. If your child is at school when you receive the diagnosis, speak with their teachers and any special education staff to work out a comprehensive support plan that will assist their learning and interaction with other students.

11. **Get organised** and find a handy place to keep all of your child's medical records and reports, where you can access them easily and quickly if need be. You will often end up on waiting lists to access different interventions, or have to leave phone messages for specialists. Hence, you should be able to pull out all necessary paperwork at a moment's notice.

    It's also a good idea to maintain some kind of informal diary on your child's progress when they start different therapies, so you can track how well they are responding, the success of outcomes and whether things might need to be revised in any way. This is useful for reviewing any interventions with your therapy team.

12. **Maintain a sense of humour!** My ability to laugh at myself and at life has got me through many a difficult situation and anxious moment. It's easy to throw ourselves a pity party once in a while when confronted with various challenges, and particularly when we have a really bad day.

    But laughter really is the best medicine. One of the most valuable lessons we can teach Autistic children, who are about 80% more likely to be bullied than their neurotypical peers, is to not take themselves, other people's opinions or life in general too seriously.

13. **Don't stop believing!** I know, it sounds very Glee Club, but while this might seem like a tired cliché; it's actually very sage advice.

    So what should you believe in? Yourself, your child and the love you have for them. Nothing else really matters when all is said and done, right? This is your special little person, with his or her own life experiences to live each day.

As parents, it's up to us to support and teach our children; allowing them to journey their own unique path through life as we demonstrate with our actions and words, what it means to be a compassionate and decent human being.

Remember, Autism is a word associated with those of us who possess a different way of processing the world. It does not define the individual, and neither should we.

6. DISCLOSING A DIAGNOSIS – SHARING WITH FAMILY, FRIENDS AND OTHERS

Who, when and how you share an Autism diagnosis will be entirely dependent on you and your family. Many members of your 'inner circle' will no doubt be aware of your child's differences and might even already acknowledge their Autistic traits.

It becomes trickier when you are dealing with people who are not so familiar with your child or your family, and in particular, new people you encounter along your journey – as your child begins pre-school and transitions into new social settings for instance.

Sharing with siblings
How you inform a child's brother or sister of their Autism will be influenced by their age. If you are explaining why Jack cannot talk or why he interacts differently during play to a toddler, keep it simple with comments like, "Jack thinks a little bit differently, so he can find it a bit harder to do some things."

Six to eight year olds will comprehend a little more detail, like; "Jack has Autism, which means his brain works a bit differently. So sometimes he finds it hard to play with toys the same way you do, or he loves trains so much that he always likes to tell us about them."

Importantly, try to avoid defining your child entirely by their Autism or making them seem remarkable to their siblings, by pointing out we are all alike in that we are all very different. And teach them that Autism doesn't mean their brother or sister is 'broken'.

You can get some great picture books to explain Autistic differences for these age groups. For older kids and teenagers, you can talk to their sibling's specific behaviours and traits, in context of the Autistic experience in a world that favours social and cultural conformity above diversity.

Sharing with the school community
Teachers and school staff are so exposed to children on the Spectrum within their classrooms these days that most of them will probably suspect your child's diagnosis long before you speak to them about it.

Some parents are concerned that if they disclose at school, their child will be a more likely target for bullies and staff could treat them differently.

However, if you intend to put your child through the mainstream education system, chances are they will need some type of support at various stages. Hence it will be necessary to share the diagnosis so that suitable resources can be allocated to them to assist in their learning and classroom interactions.

A general, guided classroom discussion can be arranged to talk about your child's diagnosis if you have concerns about their peers singling them out. This can be focused on a theme of 'diversity', where all students are asked to list their strengths and weaknesses and complete various self-awareness exercises to highlight their own unique talents and nuances.

Sharing with the wider community

Sometimes it can be beneficial and necessary to disclose your child's diagnosis to various members of the community.

Trusted neighbours can be useful allies on the Autism journey, particularly if meltdowns can be overly loud and prolonged. Likewise, if your child tends to leave the family home unsupervised or wander away, it can be of benefit for trusted people in your community to be informed about their diagnosis, as well as their unique traits, behaviours and sensory/anxiety triggers.

A US based study found that around half of all children on the Spectrum between the ages of four and ten will 'elope' or 'abscond' (as it's commonly referred to) at some stage, which is four times more than for non-Autistic children.

If your child is at risk of wandering off, it can also pay to speak with local police about their Autistic characteristics, any distinct behaviours and the best way to approach them so they do not feel threatened or in danger, as well as who to contact in the event of such a situation.

Sharing with your child

Many parents have asked me when and how they should inform their child about their Autism diagnosis. We decided it was imperative to give Aislinn a context for her feelings and differences as soon as she was capable of understanding.

Of course our situation is perhaps a little unique, in that I have always talked to her about her Asperger's in relation to my own Autistic experience.

How and when to disclose your child's diagnosis is obviously a consideration to be made at each parents' own discretion, and will depend on the child themselves.

I personally believe withholding this information from your child indefinitely can be detrimental to their growth in the long term. To begin with, an unwillingness to openly discuss what it is that makes your child different will send them a message that those differences are somehow wrong or bad.

They will most likely feel confused about who they are and why they are not like 'other children' they interact with, which can lead to feelings of insecurity and self-doubt – who am I and where do I fit it, or why can't I fit in?

On the other hand, openly and confidently discussing your child's diagnosis will give them a greater insight into who they are and why they process the world differently to their peers.

Again, make sure the conversation is around their collective strengths and weaknesses and demonstrate to them that we are all unique in our own ways, by sharing your own qualities of character – the ones you're proud of and the ones you work on every day.

Understanding goes a long way in developing a child's self-awareness - arguably the best gift you can give an Autistic child, because with self-awareness comes a greater capacity to learn how to self-regulate, self-advocate and manage our own needs – which is critical to shaping a future of independence.

If you are uncertain, or need guidance around how and when to broach this important conversation with your child, seek assistance from a qualified counsellor or specialist.

A final word

Remember, an Autism diagnosis isn't the end. Rather, it heralds the beginning of your family's journey into a brave new world. This will be a life that challenges you on many occasions, testing your patience and resolve. There will be highs and lows, laughter and tears. It won't be the easiest path, but no one ever said life was meant to be easy. What I can tell you is that this journey will be worth every minute!

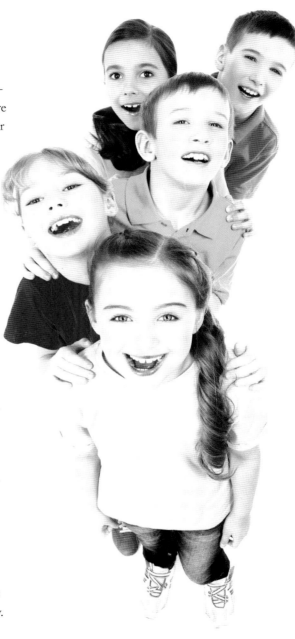

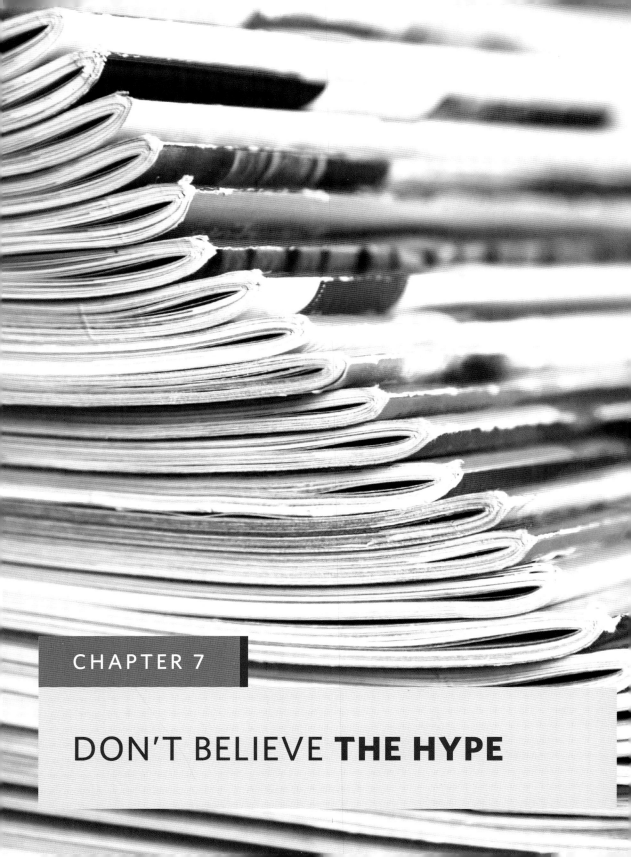

CHAPTER 7

DON'T BELIEVE **THE HYPE**

One of the most contentious issues surrounding Autism is how it's portrayed and perceived across the world, with many negative associations and stereotypes attached to the label.

This stigma comes from a culture of pathologising the Autistic experience, to the point where we have been reduced to arguments about whether it's okay to refer to people as 'Autistic', or whether we should use 'person first" language – i.e. "a person with Autism."

Ironically, those who most often debate the complexities of defining Autism appropriately are usually non-Autistic people attempting to be politically correct. However, this dialogue actually highlights all of the historical social prejudices associated with the word 'Autistic'.

Logically, to imply that someone might be offended if we call him or her Autistic is to imply that Autism in itself is offensive. That's why I question the need for some Autistic people to say, "My Autism doesn't define me."

What if it did? Would that be such a bad thing? It's an integral mechanic of your brain function and given that the brain controls our entire life force, perhaps it does go some way to defining you.

> If I could snap my fingers and be non-Autistic, I would not. Autism is part of what I am.

TEMPLE GRANDIN

However, the Autistic stigma should not! The experience of an 'Autistic' or neuro-atypical person is just as unique, and therefore exactly the same as, the experience of a 'normal' or 'neurotypical' person.

A COMMUNITY DIVIDED – BUT WHY?

The Autism community itself is all at sea when it comes to what Autistic difference represents. Some claim it's an absolute disability that they would gladly 'cure' themselves, or their offspring of, if given the chance.

Then there are those (like myself), who feel it represents a different way of processing and interacting with the world – not less than, just different.

The many unfavourable stigmas associated with the word 'Autism' can challenge and ultimately change the way parents look at, and interact with our children. The pathology of Autism impinges on the natural, nurturing relationship we have with the special little people in our lives.

We often question our parenting skills and feel adrift and alone in knowing how to raise our Autistic child to the best of our ability. As with any parent/child relationship though, if you acknowledge your child as your best teacher you will learn how to safely guide them along their path, as they grow into their own person.

I'm not saying any of this to deflate anyone's confidence in his or her parenting capacity. I just know from experience that the Autism label and its associated symptoms, cause us to relate differently to Autistic people than we perhaps would in a world that's more

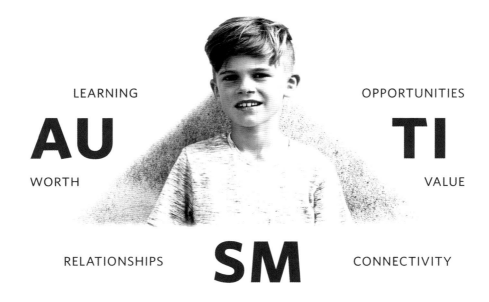

LEARNING

OPPORTUNITIES

AU

TI

WORTH

VALUE

RELATIONSHIPS

SM

CONNECTIVITY

Do we have the right to rob our children of the opportunity to grow and develop into their own unique potential? No one's personal journey should be restricted to the confines of three little syllables.

accepting of neurodiversity. And that's something we should all reflect on.

AUTISM – A SOCIAL DISABILITY?

When you start peeling away the stigmas, the question then has to be asked; how much of the Autistic experience actually represents inherent disability? And how much is social disability?

If lived in another context – where difference makes no difference and everyone was afforded the opportunity to be our own (unique) 'normal' –Autism would not necessarily be pathologised, and the Autistic experience reduced to a list of incapacities.

The term Autism Spectrum Disorder (ASD) is based on a narrow pathology definition that's contributed to the

systematic marginalization of 'neurodivergents' throughout the ages.

The notion that Autistic people have a 'disorder' should have been thrown out with the same bathwater that saw Autism diagnosed as a form of mental illness, like schizophrenia, in the 1900s. Both views are archaic and have no basis in scientific evidence.

Worryingly, such biases are causing the fundamental needs of Autistic people to be overlooked in favour of heavily funded research that seeks to identify 'cause and cure'.

Not so long ago, homosexuality was perceived as a disease too. It's no coincidence that the Autistic pride movement has some striking similarities to the gay pride movement. In this world, difference has become a disability.

AUTISM AS THE ENEMY OF SOCIAL ORDER

Think I'm being alarmist, or exaggerating the extent of the damage Autistic stereotypes inflict?

While writing this book, six people were tragically killed in Santa Barbara (USA). The 22-year-old perpetrator, Elliot Rodger was widely reported in the media as being Autistic.

Even though studies have shown that Autistic people are no more prone to violent criminal acts than non-Autistic people (in fact they are more likely to be the target of these crimes) - the "Autism" excuse has become a common media go to.

As a community, we should be asking why Autism is apparently such an easy target to blame for someone choosing to commit a socially intolerable act?

If we ever hope to truly address and stamp out things like the Santa Barbara tragedy, we must consider why crime occurs from a bigger picture perspective and broader social context. The answers are not to be found in simplifying the reasoning by blaming a word and its stereotypes.

Autism has become a common scapegoat for various social issues. You will rarely see Autism discussed for its potential and possibility – for what the Autistic individual could contribute to the world around them - but rather the level of drain Autism places on our various social systems, i.e. education, justice, welfare, etc.

Papers and studies around 'expected outcomes' for those on the Autism Spectrum paint a bleak and frankly disheartening picture, trotting out statistics to suggest a future of:

1. Low educational attainment
2. Low employment
3. Reduced living independence
4. Reduced social functioning
5. Reduced potential to be in a successful long-term relationship.

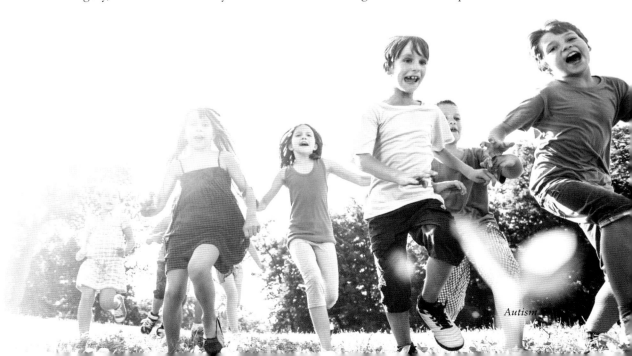

Autism

7. WHY THE AUTISM STIGMA EXISTS – LABELLING DIFFERENT

The World Health Organization says Autistic people are a "vulnerable group", often subjected to stigma and discrimination, including unjust deprivation of health and education services, and opportunities to engage and participate in their communities.

Restricted access to these essential community relationships and supports creates unnecessary emotional, economic and care burdens on Autistic people and their families and as such, we find that these negative perceptions run in a self-perpetuating cycle that looks something like this:

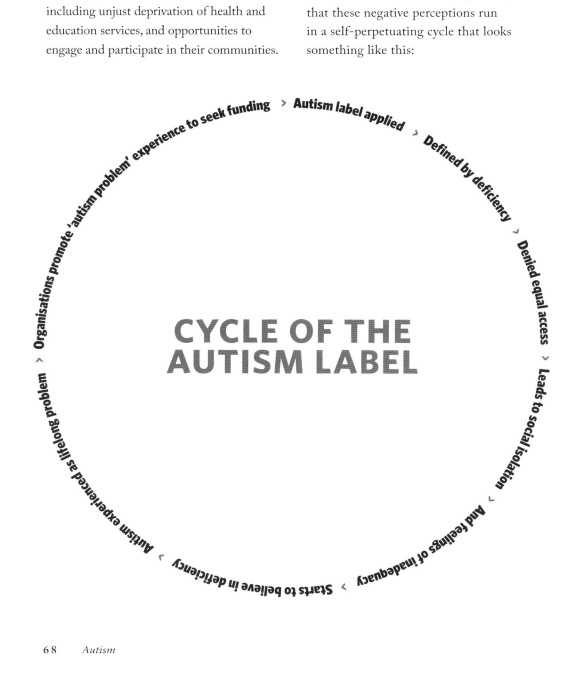

CYCLE OF THE AUTISM LABEL

Autism label applied > Defined by deficiency > Denied equal access > Leads to social isolation > And feelings of inadequacy > Starts to believe in deficiency > Autism experienced as lifelong problem > Organisations promote 'autism problem' experience to seek funding > Autism label applied

Autism's deficiency stigmas are defined and subsequently "treated" according to the person's apparent inability to conform to society's ever-narrowing yardstick of normal. But does one's capacity to conform and toe the 'normal' line actually align with their overall wellbeing or life purpose?

I would argue that conforming to perceptions of normalcy is in direct conflict with attaining a state of harmony and balance in this world for anyone, let alone the Autistic person.

Your best and healthiest you will look entirely different to my best and healthiest me. Not just because I have Asperger's and you may not, but because our life journey's will never be the same. That's the beauty of humanity and the reason we are able to evolve.

Imagine if the cavemen had accepted cave dwelling as 'normal'. One day a caveman comes along who challenges that perception. But instead of listening to this different way of thinking, the others in his tribe decide he is mentally unstable and either ostracise or try to 'cure' his 'psychosis'. Perhaps we would still be cave dwellers today.

What would happen if the Autism gene was eliminated from the gene pool?

You would have a bunch of people standing around in a cave, chatting and socializing and not getting anything done.

TEMPLE GRANDIN

NORMAL IS A FOUR-LETTER WORD

The notion that there is one kind of 'normal', which defines us all as human beings, is ludicrous. Not to mention completely boring!

When we recognise that 'normal' is simply each person's own state of mind, then maybe we can stop insisting that everyone's mind should work in the same way and start celebrating the potential of minds that can do lots of different things.

My normal way of learning might not be in a classroom surrounded by other children my own age, where conformity is valued over creativity. My normal way of socialising might not be looking you in the eye and adopting niceties for the sake of polite social pretence. My normal relationships might not involve constantly reaffirming another person's value in my life, because they cannot acknowledge their own self-worth.

But guess what? It's still my 'normal'. Or maybe we should start saying…it's my different. Imagine a world without 'normal' and all its limiting expectations.

This is change we would all benefit from embracing and committing to – restoring everyone's right to truly be themselves, experiencing life through their own realised potential and possibility…a world in which we are truly free.

The discrimination all too often experienced by Autistic people is entirely unnecessary when we recognise that as human beings, we are all, in some way, shape or form, distinctive – even if we reduce that down to a fingerprint.

My somewhat convoluted point is that the word 'normal' should be discarded in the context of humanity, so that Autistic people are not incessantly traumatised by a series of therapists and systems that seek to stifle their truth and 'normalise' them.

I believe it's time to rethink Autism, and redefine 'normal'. Instead of trying to cram every personality into one standard package with a few unique souls who "think outside the box", let's do away with the 'boxes', giving people an opportunity to spread their differently coloured wings and define their own life experience.

Maybe rather than trying to make everyone 'fit in', we can acknowledge that it's okay for anyone to 'stand out'. When we get to that point, then perhaps we can start to explore alternative ways to accommodate diversity in our schools, workplaces and society, until difference makes no difference and everyone is afforded the same rights and opportunities.

8. THE IMPACT OF THE AUTISM STIGMA ON INDIVIDUALS AND FAMILIES

When we pronounce someone Autistic by comparing their differences to a perception of 'normal' (as defined by 'the majority'), and then deem those differences inadequate, we are telling them that unless they change who they are in order to accommodate expectations, they will never be accepted.

We take away the person's identity before they have a chance to uncover their own potential – insisting that they learn how to be more like everybody else, instead of who they truly are.

Self-discovery is a vital aspect of human growth. Embarking on our own personal journey gives us the chance to learn about ourselves, including our likes and dislikes, our strengths and vulnerabilities and our own unique talents and character.

When we are inhibited on this journey, we start to question who we are and our life's purpose, leading to insecurity and feelings of worthlessness.

This loss of identity, along with the underlying stigmas that contaminate a person's self-awareness and how others relate to them, can cause the Autistic person to experience life as a series of traumatic events.

Would the Autistic child be bullied as a 'weak target' if Autism was perceived as a strength of character? Or if different ways of processing the world were acknowledged and validated, rather than labelled and marginalised?

Would barriers to mainstream schooling and employment for Autistic people be so prevalent if these systems did not have such a rigid intolerance of difference, in favour of conformity? Or if there were no preconceived ideas about how the person would perform and function academically, socially and productively (based on a 'limitation' understanding of Autism)?

When we tell a person that unless they can pass as 'normal', they will forever be seen as some kind of problem to be fixed, and when we refer to Autism as a social burden, we undermine the value of the Autistic individual's life.

Ironically, the very Autistic stigmas that suggest we are incapable of relating to people, actually create barriers to 'normal' social interaction. The insidious perceptions of Autism in our world cause others to approach us from a place of bias.

Whether consciously or unconsciously, judgments are made as to our capacity to hold a conversation and maintain relationships, creating very real obstacles to healthy human expression as expectations limit the potential for a meaningful exchange between the Autistic person and non-Autistic person.

Being constantly reminded that you are different and have no place among 'normal' society isolates Autistic people and their families, displacing them and suggesting that they will never 'belong' unless they can 'fit in'.

It creates crippling and yes, disabling insecurities, with the person's self-awareness based on weakness and limitation above strength and potential.

> Children with ASD can grow beyond their limitations and develop into wonderful, productive citizens. All we have to do is see through those limitations to the bright kids they really are, helping them past their difficulties without allowing them to be labelled and restricted by their diagnoses.

KARINA POIRIER

9. HOW YOUR ATTITUDE TO AUTISM CAN CHANGE THE WORLD

So how do we address these misconceptions and stereotypes? How do we ensure that every Autistic individual has the right and opportunity to reach their full potential in a world of true awareness and acceptance?

First we take back the label, and redefine it based on our own experiences. We share our stories and come out of isolation to acknowledge that even if it looks different, we each have a part to play in this thing called 'life'.

We stop allowing stereotypes and their associated expectations to define who we are and how we contribute to the world. We acknowledge that every life has purpose and value. And we afford everyone the same right to define his or her own purpose and value.

Remember, this is your unique path of self-discovery; Autism might teach you more about yourself than you ever imagined possible. I love it when I speak to families about their children and they say, "I have grown so much as a person because of my child's Autism." Or, "Autism has made me a better person." Those words are beautiful music to my ears and have so much power!

Importantly, don't give your power to the stereotypes and stigmas. When you are fatigued and frustrated by how difficult 'difference' can be in a world that celebrates 'normal', reach out to support from within our community. Seek out others who can empathise with your experiences and will not judge you for having a 'bad day'.

It's also important to have respite options in place. This can be tricky depending on the level of care your child requires and available resources in the community, but without a break every now and then it's more likely you will slip into feelings of negativity and anxiety.

Ultimately, the only way we will combat unfavourable Autistic stereotypes is to become pro-active in our efforts to create a more understanding world.

Why we all need to become Autism Advocates

Our community is rich in knowledge, compassion and determination. As a collective, we have the potential, the knowledge and the resources to effect real change; affording every human being the right and opportunity to discover, nurture and experience their own life's purpose.

Next time someone tells you that your child has Autism, so they must not have much empathy or imagination, remind them that it's today's society that's actually lacking in these qualities, not your child.

You only need to look at widely held notions of how children should be educated to realise how inflexible, uninspired and unimaginative society has become in its perceptions of 'normal'.

Changing an ingrained belief about any sort of minority group is no easy feat. But for the sake of our children and generations to come, someone has to start somewhere. And I think the best place to start is from within.

It's up to us – Autistic adults, parents of Autistic children, the peak bodies and support groups and the academics who have studied us long enough to know that different does not mean "less than" – to acknowledge that this is our battle.

We must rise to the challenge – not of raising an Autistic child or being Autistic - but of addressing the inherent social issues of our time that have shaped a world in which capitalist ideals are pitting human beings against one another and dividing us all.

We must focus our energy on building and sustaining a connected community, so that we can channel our efforts into finding a better world – which values human compassion and connection - rather than fighting a broken one.

Consider Autism a friend rather than a foe and you might be surprised what you and your child are capable of. The alternative is simply a waste of time, because Autism is a part of your life. Here are a few of my tips to make Autism your family's friend:

1. Remind yourself every day how wonderful your family is and the blessings that are your children.
2. Count the good things you have in your life and celebrate the triumphs.
3. Learn from your mistakes and move ahead with your newfound knowledge, rather than dwelling on them.
4. Smile and laugh – your energy will influence a lot of what is going on for your child, so remaining calm, happy and positive will help them immensely.
5. Teach yourself how to shine from within, so you can show your child that we all have an inner light to share with the world.

6. Let go of expectations about who your child should become or what they should be when they 'grow up'. Instead teach them to live in the moment, rather than worrying about tomorrow.

The biggest and most challenging change we need to make

Perhaps the most impressive rethink around stigmatised differences like Autism will occur when we acknowledge that the world, not Autistic people, needs fixing.

So long as we live in a global village that puts profits above people and promotes a competitive, capitalist way of life that's unforgiving and "dog eat dog", social injustices like those Autism stigmas perpetuate will continue to corrupt the true human experience of connection and compassion that we are most naturally attuned to.

Rather than forcing Autistic people to cope with a world that's cruel and unforgiving, why do we not, as a collective, strive to make the world a less confronting and callous reality?

Before you buy into the need for your child to undergo extensive therapies so they "learn to be normal" one day, perhaps you should stop to consider whether the world's 'normality' is really worth challenging your child's perceptions of self to the point where they struggle with a lack of identity.

Many therapists and well paid experts for whom Autism (as a burden of disease to be fixed) pays the bills, will suggest that Autistic people are at risk of 'not belonging' if they cannot be programmed to conform.

I would suggest that the lack of identity experienced when we are forced to be something that's not a true reflection of self, is what causes us to feel as though we don't belong in this world.

So before you worry about treating your child to bring them closer to normal, perhaps you should take a moment to ask yourself, "Is this world's current definition of normal really the most I would want for my child?"

> Autists are the ultimate square pegs, and the problem with pounding a square peg into a round hole is not that the hammering is hard work. It's that you're destroying the peg.

PAUL COLLINS

10. AUTISTIC PEOPLE SHOW US EVERY DAY - DIFFERENT IS NOT DEFICIENT

Of course there are varying degrees of the Autistic experience and associated disability. Non-verbal communicators obviously have more challenges to overcome as they navigate a world where speech is most commonly used, for instance.

However, even some of the more profound Autistic disabilities, where individuals are non-verbal or appear 'shut off', should not be the basis of prejudiced assumptions around how a person experiences life.

Someone's ability or inability to speak

does not necessarily determine their ability to think or feel. These are distinct neural processes. Wrapping them all up in 'the Autistic' package and suggesting that being a non-verbal communicator somehow reduces a person's potential for a meaningful life in every aspect, is completely unwarranted and unfair.

In recent times, modern technology has given Autistic people who are non-verbal access to augmentative communication devices in the form of mobile tablets, like iPads, specialist apps and software.

While "assisted communication" has sparked controversial debate around whether people are actually "speaking for themselves", many of the very personal messages delivered via this alternative form of expression suggest that non-verbal Autistic people have been misrepresented and misunderstood for far too long.

Blowing many long-held stigmas out of the proverbial water, the capacity of non-verbal people on the Autism Spectrum to, not only type full words and sentences, but also express their desire for communication with deep and insightful musings was brought to the world's attention with the 2010 release of a book called 'The Golden Hat – Talking Back to Autism'.

Kate Winslet put her name to the book, which features some of the UK actress's high profile celebrity friends, and subsequently co-founded the British and US based Golden Hat Foundation as an Autism ambassador – to "honour the intellectual capabilities of people with Autism".

One of the children who featured in the book was twelve year old Kell Thorsteinsson, a nonverbal Autistic boy who had just learnt to communicate with a letterboard. He composed the following, moving poem:

THE GOLDEN HAT
This boy had a golden hat.
The hat was magical. It could talk.
The boy did not have any voice.
He had Autism.
His hat was always with him.
His hat was lost one day.
Now he had no way of telling
them his stories.
His mom and dad became sad.
They taught him spelling on a letterboard.
It was hard.

A few years ago, American teen Carly Fleischmann astounded the world with her own unique message about the non-verbal Autistic experience of life. Appearing on various US television shows, including Ellen DeGeneres, Carly demonstrated that communicating from one's soul isn't restricted to the spoken word.

Mothers have shared stories with me about various medical experts presuming their nonverbal child is intellectually disabled, only to one day find they start speaking or communicating with augmentative technology, and displaying high levels of intelligence and perception.

One of my dear friends decided to homeschool all three of her Autistic children after her daughter was repeatedly bullied at school and teachers and the principle disregarded her non-verbal son as being incapable of learning.

They advised her his tested IQ was below 70 and that she should essentially have no expectation for any real progress during his academic years. They decided he was incapable of learning.

A few years later at the age of ten, her son was studying Year 12 Physics and Maths and had immersed himself in the world of computer programming language – his passionate obsession.

We cannot presume that because a child is non-verbal, they are incapable of experiencing a meaningful life.

11. AUTISM AND INTELLECTUAL AND LEARNING DISABILITIES

About a year ago I watched a life changing video. It was a presentation in which the speaker told his audience that there are some 70 plus ways of learning. Only one of them is verbal.

However, all of our modern education systems are based on verbal learning.

Statistics suggest that almost half (46%) of children identified with Autism have average to above average intellectual ability. Between 44 to 52% are thought to have a learning disability. However, findings that suggest up to half of all people on the Autism Spectrum have a lower than average IQ are still considered inconclusive.

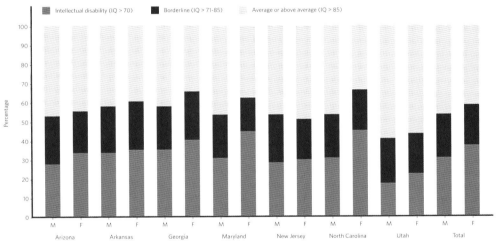

Abbreviations: ASD = Autism Spectrum Disorder, F = female, IQ = Intelligence Quotient, M = Male
*Includes sites that has intellectual ability data available for >70% of children who met the ASD case definition.

Most recent intelligence quotient (IQ) as of age 8 years among children identified with Autism spectrum disorder (ASD) for whom test data were available*, by site and sex

AUTISM AND DEVELOPMENTAL DISABILITIES MONITORING NETWORK, SEVEN SITES†, UNITED STATES, 2010

Current schooling institutions and applications across places like the UK, America and Australia do not favour diversity. Compliance and conformity are the order of the day in classrooms where everyone is expected to learn in one certain way and at the same common pace, without any thought for individuality. And certainly no flexibility to accommodate individual differences.

Even though it has been demonstrated in various studies that (many, but certainly not all) Autistic children are generally visual and/or kinetic learners, due to their unique neurodiversity, we continue to teach them within the context and expectations of "normalcy".

Perhaps if these rigid education systems were to bend a little, demonstrating the very flexibility of thought that we suggest Autistic people are lacking, some of the more common learning disabilities associated with Autism – dyslexia and dyspraxia for instance – would be less of an impediment to the acquisition of knowledge.

A FINAL WORD

When we create labels for people, based on a perceived deviation from recognised social and cultural constructs of 'normal', we assert an insidious and pervasive kind of control over their life, which can in turn alienate them from their truth.

I believe this is what causes so much of the human distress and dis-ease we see in today's world – this alienation of the person from their own awareness of self. On some level, we eventually realise that we are not living our true life's purpose...the one thing that has the potential to make us truly happy.

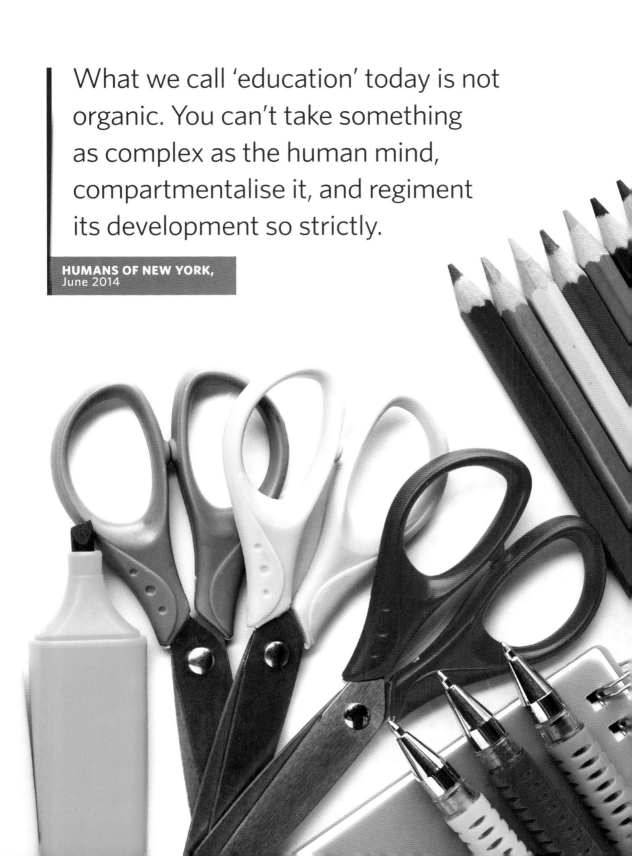

What we call 'education' today is not organic. You can't take something as complex as the human mind, compartmentalise it, and regiment its development so strictly.

HUMANS OF NEW YORK,
June 2014

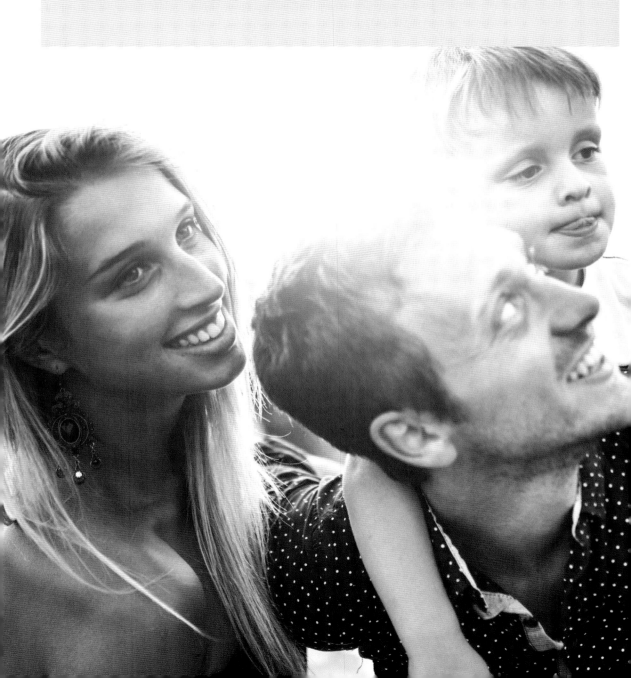

CHAPTER 8

LIVING BEYOND THE LABELS

Whilst in the middle of writing this book, as often happens in our over-loaded modern lives, our family's path suddenly took a very sharp turn into the unknown.

The scary kind of unknown where Reilly, our three year old, became increasingly sick with ketoacidosis, before being air-lifted to hospital and diagnosed with Type 1 Diabetes. His system was shutting down; with such elevated blood sugars the levels were unreadable.

I had noticed numerous warning signs over the two or so weeks leading up to the July 3 incident, voicing my concerns to more than one person, including a random doctor from the medical clinic we normally attend.

Our little man ended up in hospital on that fateful Thursday, after a preceding appointment with the GP who had seen him only once before (our usual family doctor was unavailable).

I explained the worrying symptoms and events that had brought us to the clinic. Reilly was drinking more, urinating with extreme frequency (I told him of 150 plus visits to the toilet within a five hour period alone on the weekend prior), increasing lethargy, weight loss and irritability.

During our one previous dealing with this particular doctor, he very quickly referred to our family history of Autism, suggesting we should take Reilly for an assessment regarding his apparent 'delayed speech'.

He was about 20 months old at the time, with a few distinct words and at that stage I certainly wasn't concerned. Besides which, the reason for our consul-tation back then had nothing to do with Autism, but rather an issue of recurring conjunctivitis.

Fast forward some sixteen months later (Reilly now exhibits an extensive vocabulary for his age) and here we were again; same doctor with seemingly the same shortsighted approach to diagnostic practice.

Instead of immediately exploring an organic reason for Reilly's latest disquieting symptoms, the doctor stated with authority, "It could be THE AUTISM. You haven't had him assessed yet?"

I politely answered his apprehensions around 'the Autism' – yes; he admittedly has some 'Autistic' traits and tendencies, including various sensory responses. However, while there are a few possible signs, labelling his neuro-divergence was really not my priority at that particular moment.

Autism won't make my son physically ill, I explained to the GP, with diminishing patience.

Long story short, 'Dr No Idea' sent us away to contemplate a referral to the paedi-atrician for an Autism assessment. Oh, and just in case something organic was going on, a specimen jar accompanied with vague instructions; "Just get a sample and take it into your local pathology lab when you have some time."

This doctor's judgement was so clouded by a perception of 'the Autism' that he failed to see a critically ill child (barely capable of) standing in front of him.

This is the problem with labelling a difference like Autism. Firstly, Autism isn't going to kill my son. I know that many tragic circumstances have resulted in the loss of beautiful Autistic souls for various indirect reasons.

But Autism isn't a life threatening illness. It doesn't require us to inject our child with insulin twice a day so he can survive, or constantly make his fingers bleed to assess his glucose levels.

In this instance, it was the medical perceptions of 'normal' behaviour and development, aligned with the pathologising and subsequent stigmatization of Autism, which could indeed have cost our little boy's life. If I had not been so insistent on them investigating further just two days later, I hate to think what the outcome might have been.

We have a new difference to acclimatise to in our household. It's Type 1 Diabetes. While some might perceive Autism as a heartbreaking, debilitating tragedy, I know we won't have to wake every hour to make sure our 'Autistic' children are still breathing. And Autism doesn't increase the likelihood of your child one day requiring a new kidney, or losing a foot or their eyesight.

The difference with this difference is that I would gladly cure T1. But innately different brain functions like Autism? Well, one day an Autistic person might just find the T1 cure that our little man needs…you never know.

12. FOCUS ON THE PERSON, NOT THE LABEL

The point of sharing this story with you is to demonstrate that everything is about perspective. Our family is fortunate enough to have a different view of different and an understanding of neurodivergence in our home that stems from years of personal life experience.

But if we had approached our children's Autism with fear and sorrow, imagine how much more deeply we would feel that apprehension when presented with this latest difference.

Instead of giving in to those initial feelings of hopelessness, grief and fear, I recognised that if Reilly was to have the quality of life he deserved and exactly the same opportunities to grow into his own person as his siblings, we had to "normalise" this thing called diabetes, for his sake.

Once again, we were being challenged to recognise that one aspect of a person's entire being is just that. Who our children are, who they will become and what direction their path takes them on, is determined by so much more than a loaded (pathologised) label, or lifelong medical condition.

Look at all of the money poured into finding a reason and remedy for Autism every year; money that could help to cure childhood cancer, Cystic Fibrosis and yes, juvenile diabetes – those far too prevalent life threatening conditions where increasingly desperate patients pray for cures.

While I believe the Autism community is deserving of assistance, right now most of the 'help' offered by those controlling funding in this sector is a persistent attempt to make everyone fit the perception of 'normal'.

Where are the initiatives designed to truly acknowledge and integrate difference into our community? The initiatives that focus on the person first, not the pathologising of Autism as a label, which ultimately leads to that one-size-fits-all approach that we know doesn't work.

Where are the initiatives that seek to advocate for and create equality in our world around the Autistic experience? What about schools and places of employment where people are not required to fit in, but encouraged to develop into their own person?

This is what I would like to see money being spent on. More individualistic approaches to the challenges Autism can present in our world of 'normal', and ways we can better accommodate the neurally divergent who walk among us.

So our youngest now has a label of his own. But I can tell you that it will not be allowed to encompass, envelop and eventually be the only thing that defines him in this world.

He is still our little man and that's what matters most – he is still here with us, to love and nurture. We are blessed with this beautiful, different soul in our lives.

As parents we have a responsibility to our children, to accept them for who they are. When we get caught up in labels and stigmas, largely based on perceptions from a world that doesn't understand (and fears that which it doesn't know), we are approaching our children from our own place of fear and uncertainty.

If you let him or her, every child born into this world will tell you who he or she is, at that very innate level. It's up to us to listen and respond accordingly.

> I know of nobody who is purely Autistic, or purely neurotypical. Even God has some Autistic moments, which is why the planets spin.
>
> **JERRY NEWPORT**

Labelling versus enabling

According to the dictionary definition, to enable means to:

- make able; give power, means, competence, or ability to; authorise
- make possible or easy
- make ready; equip

Parents begin enabling our children from the moment they are born. Our role, by its very nature, is as our child's enabler in their formative years. As they are learning about the world around them and importantly, who they are as they journey through it, we are meant to empower them; with sufficient knowledge of self and the resulting confidence in all they do.

Aside from protecting them fiercely, this is our purpose as parents. We are not meant to 'mould' our children's minds – this is a process that evolves naturally if a child is allowed to explore and retain that instinctive curiosity that compels them to learn in every moment.

It's our job to encourage the innate 'need to know' they are born with. This is positive enabling – something that can prove challenging in a world that urges us, as parents, to teach our children how to conform, compete and consume; all at the expense of that gorgeous, natural curiosity.

When your child receives an Autism diagnosis, the stigmas all come crashing in on top of it, reinforced by misguided and negative information from all corners.

When you start labelling your child, you effectively replace this positive type of enabling with a form co-dependence, based on a perception of incapacity.

They start to learn about themselves from a different perspective. Remember, you would have been informed (most likely in your child's presence) that he or she has inflexibility of thought, lack of imagination and empathy, and significant cognitive, social and behavioural developmental delays.

With the application of the Autism label in such a negative foundation, we immediately risk not only stifling a child's true personhood, but also changing the nature of our relationship with them.

We lose sight of our nurturing role and how very important it is and get caught up in trying to find 'answers' to improve their lot in life. Ironically, the person with the answers is standing right in front of us – because our children will teach us who they are and what they need from us as positive enablers, if we are willing to drop our pre-conceived ideas and expectations and just pay attention.

When we begin to enable based on stigmas associated with labels such as Autism, we inadvertently exert a negative influence over our child's development.

Some parents feel the need to respond with a medley of therapeutic approaches in an attempt to 'cure' their child's Autism, while others make accommodations in the family home based on the assumption that their child is unable to learn and develop 'normally'.

By doing so, we are removing that positive enabling influence that seeks to empower our children's natural development according to their own ability and perception of self, with an approach that tells them something is 'wrong' with the person they are.

Often parents who choose to enable their children positively will do things a bit differently. They don't feel the need to 'over-therapise' their child, dragging them from appointment to appointment in a bid to 'fix them'.

Instead they will engage in play based approaches and accept that their child will or will not talk when they are ready and able. That perhaps not every single one of us is designed to develop, function and communicate in the exact same way.

When you let go of the labels – and I'm talking 'normal' as much as I'm talking 'Autism' now - you become that positive enabling force in your child's world.

> If you're treading quicksand in the swamp of what-might- have-been, you can be sure that's the message your child gets. You're a rare person if being constantly reminded of your shortcomings spurs you to improve. For the rest of us, it's a self-esteem squasher. Time to grab for that overhead vine and realise that only a pencil dot separates "bitter" and "better.

ELLEN NOTBOHM

Enabling your child's own definition of the Autistic experience

While it's necessary to recognise your child's Autism as an integral aspect of their true self, it's also necessary to allow them to define their own Autistic experience in this world.

It's tough to do this as a parent, because we all want to protect our children and make sure they never get hurt. But it's essential if we want them to not just survive, but also thrive in their own unique way.

So what does that entail? Well, in no particular order…

1. Refusing to limit your child's potential based on a diagnosis that indicates they are different.

2. Taking a moment to really acknowledge that "fitting in" doesn't necessarily entail "doing what everyone else does".

3. Allowing your child to discover their own self and walk their own journey.

4. Seeking out any supports they need in order to successfully manage the above, including Autistic mentors who can decrease their feelings of isolation and encourage self-confidence in acknowledging and accepting who they are.

And of course, it means recognising that "your Autistic child" is still simply "your child", just as they were before diagnosis; with all of those interesting and unique quirks and flaws that we are, each and every one of us, born with.

13. LETTING THE PERSON DEFINE WHO THEY ARE BEYOND THE LABEL OF AUTISM

If you only take one thing from this entire book, I hope it's to allow your Autistic loved one to reach for the sky and feel uninhibited by misguided and medicalised stigmas and stereotypes based on limitation.

Every child isn't a carbon copy of the one that came before and neither they should be. But when we start insisting that they tick standard boxes of development and achievement that's what we are telling them.

If you enable your child to know who they are and be empowered in that knowledge, they will stand a much better chance of successfully navigating their journey

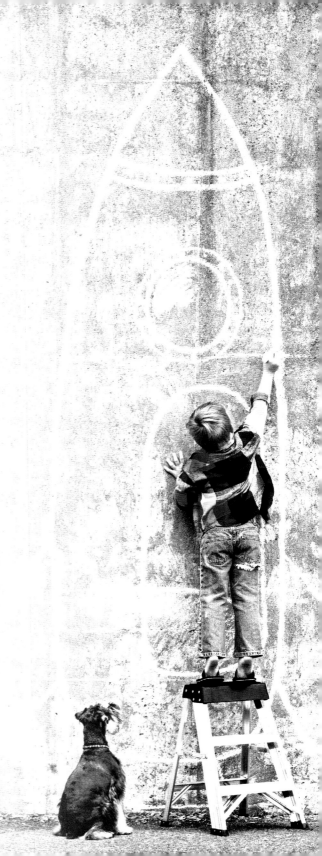

through life, confident in themselves.

This confidence will in turn give them the courage to explore and learn more of who they are and how they navigate the world. They may not do these things in a 'normal' way. In fact, chances are they will always be doing things in a way their peers consider different.

But allowing them to define their own person will be the most significant action you can take as the parent of an Autistic child, and the most precious gift you could give them.

It means they can advocate for themselves as adults, with a clear understanding of what makes them tick and what pushes their sensory buttons.

This self-awareness will have significant ramifications throughout their whole lives, particularly as they step into the world of adulthood.

Consider schooling and employment for the empowered Autistic person, who knows him or herself so well that they can effectively communicate their experiences and needs to a teacher or employer, in order to resolve a concern. They can speak of their Autism openly, without fear of condemnation or perceptions tainted by stigmas.

All it takes is telling your child, "Yes, you can", until "Yes, I can" becomes their own internal mantra, and then putting the best possible supports in place to give them every chance at success. Their own success, no one else's.

Don't think that there's a different, better child 'hiding' behind the Autism. This is your child. Love the child in front of you. Encourage his strengths, celebrate his quirks, and improve his weaknesses, the way you would with any child.

Claire Scovell LaZebnik,
author of *Growing Up on the Spectrum*

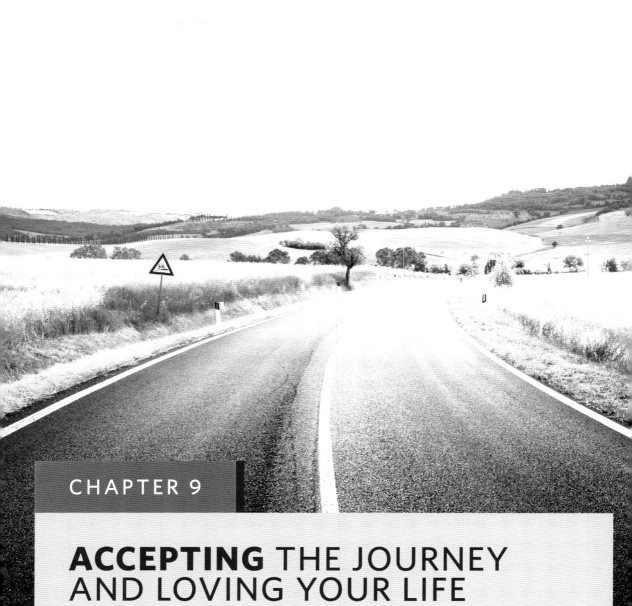

CHAPTER 9

ACCEPTING THE JOURNEY AND LOVING YOUR LIFE

Throughout my journey I have learnt a very important lesson. I don't always succeed in applying it every day mind you, because I'm human and I make my fair share of mistakes. However, it's a very good missive that I'm sure would make the world a better place if we all just did it.

You can either live life with acceptance, or with expectation.

Acceptance is a difficult road. Many things happen in life that we struggle with, because we cannot accept it has happened to us. We all process our experiences on a very personal level, right?

Something we perceive as "bad" happens and we wonder, "Why did this happen to me?"

Generally though, what we experience in one way, another is experiencing in an entirely different way. Think about the person who loses a $100 note in the street. For them it's a loss that could have great significance in their life. Now consider the person who picks up the $100, for whom finding the money could have equal, positive ramifications.

The reason we perceive things as 'bad' and take it personally, is because we have a certain expectation about our life and how it should look. We are disappointed when things are not seemingly 'perfect' – again, what perfect looks like for one person, will be entirely different to another's perfect, because it's all about perception.

When we accept things and people for what they are, we stop expecting certain results from life and from those around us.

It's a challenge, because we are taught to expect things from a very young age. We are conditioned to believe that if you get a good education, a good job immediately follows. Even on the basest level, we are told, "Be nice to people and they will be nice to you."

There is forever the suggestion that if you do X, then you can expect Y to be the outcome. But life isn't so black and white, is it? And when expectations go unmet, we feel disappointed.

The risk with expectation is that we get caught up in a cycle of self-pity and spend our days wishing things were a certain way, rather than simply dealing effectively with the cards life has dealt us in that particular moment.

By accepting, okay this has happened… you will be less likely to focus on perceived problems and more inclined to see potential solutions, before taking the necessary action to reach the most desirable outcome.

Some say acceptance means giving up control of what occurs in our world. I would argue that accepting what happens in our lives so that we can move forward and deal with it, rather than wallowing in the disappointment of unmet expectation is about self-empowerment, not abdication.

14. LEARNING TO ACCEPT YOUR LIFE WITH AUTISM

Receiving an Autism diagnosis for your child is definitely one of those tests as to whether you are living in an acceptance mindset or coming from a place of expectation.

When we received Reilly's recent diabetes diagnosis, I had the equivalent of a grief or Post Traumatic Stress response. My expectation was, "This happens to other people, not my family."

I struggled to accept it for weeks and tried to deny that this was our reality. Autism happened in our world, I could accept that, but not a critical illness.

Then I realised that if I couldn't accept this for Reilly, how was he ever going to accept it for himself? And if he failed to accept diabetes as his reality and tried to make it go away – as I longed to do - where would that leave his long-term health? In that moment, I realised I owed him acceptance.

Interestingly, my own experience of difference allowed me to accept Autism as my children's reality. That was perfectly acceptable. But that's the interesting thing about acceptance – it's much easier when we also have understanding.

Once you accept Autism as part of your journey, you will approach it from an entirely different place than you might if your perceptions are grounded in a place of unmet expectation as to how life is meant to look.

I always say Huggies commercials have a lot to answer for. Those moments on TV filled with sunshine, hugs and kisses shared by blissfully happy, rested and perfectly manicured mums and smiling bubs (all with spotless clothes), is the type of expectation the media spoon-feeds us regarding parenthood.

Once I accepted Reilly's diagnosis, I stopped asking; "Why him? Why us? Why me? Where is our perfect Huggies moment with our healthy little boy?" And I replaced that internal dialogue with a resolve and, "What now?"

My focus became about finding the best possible solution for our son and his long-term health. Furthermore, I had to recognise that the socially conditioned 'expectation' we are all taught - that "doctors are always right" – was not necessarily true. I had to instead accept their humanness, which meant that like the rest of us, they make mistakes.

When the doctors informed us that Reilly's diabetes management hinged on a high carb diet and increasingly large doses of insulin, I wasn't entirely sold.

To me this was counter-intuitive. I accepted the diagnosis and from there, determined to find the best possible approach to his treatment. Trusting my instincts, I started researching and becoming informed, in order to find a more desirable management regime that would maximise his long-term health with the right nutritional approach, whilst minimising his dependence on medical intervention.

This same philosophy of acceptance, when applied to your child's Autism diagnosis, will potentially save you a lot of time and money spent chasing 'cures' and trying therapy after therapy.

Instead of 'panic buying' when it comes to the supports you put in place for your

Autistic child, based on an expectation of who or where they should be at any given time, you are more likely to objectively weigh up the pros and cons of any suggested interventions before deciding what, if any, might be appropriate according to their desired outcomes.

Acceptance is a great way to enable and empower oneself. And the first step in your child's own journey of self-awareness and self-acceptance, is you accepting them.

Be who you are and say what you feel because those who mind don't matter and those who matter don't mind.

15. DAILY CHALLENGES & HOW TO OVERCOME THEM

Let's face it, parenting isn't an easy task and certainly comes with its fair share of trials and tribulations. We are all thrust into the role of mum or dad with less guidance than that proffered by the washing instruction tags attached to clothes.

Parenting children who do not experience ongoing anxiety and sensory issues is enough of a journey into the great unknown to make us all feel a little apprehensive, and occasionally doubt our capacity as nurturers.

The fact is all we can really do in any given moment, is the best we are capable of. We embark on a steep learning curve when children enter our world, and often I think the key to knowing what they need is to simply remember what is was to be a child ourselves.

Of course, when we are compelled to grow up and comply with the expectations of adult responsibility, recalling the many intricacies of childhood isn't an easy prospect.

When you add the additional nuances of neuro-divergence into the mix, it can make for a rather overwhelming experience of parenthood. And for parents who do not share their child's Autistic experience of the world, knowing how to manage the very different journey their child is on can be even more confronting.

Some of the more common challenges that parents may experience with regard to daily life on the Autism Spectrum include:

- Irregular sleep patterns, disturbed sleep and general insomnia,
- Extreme behavioural changes due to sensory issues and/or anxiety triggers,
- Food fussiness and food refusal, including a diet restricted to certain tastes, textures and/or colours of food, and
- Toileting anxiety and/or incontinence.

The language of behaviour
It's important to recognise and remember that whatever behaviours or issues your child is experiencing; it's not a personal affront to you as their parent. It's not the result of bad parenting per se, nor is yours a naughty, wilful or defiant child.

Rather, what you are witnessing is a physical manifestation of their experience of the world. Behaviours are a means of communicating for the child who does not quite know how to express him or herself in any other way right now.

When some type of physical or emotional trigger prompts a chemically based anxiety or fear reaction in the brain, our bodies' are programmed to kick into that instinctive fight or flight response. It 's this reactive precipice the 'Autistic' neurodivergent often sits on the edge of every day.

What makes it so difficult is that the types of differences we exhibit in this world often become the cause for our anxiety. Or should I say, the lack of acceptance and understanding of those differences.

The first step in addressing these challenges is to acknowledge this very important lesson. Then you can start to ask yourself what might be triggering these situations and work toward addressing those underlying causal effects, rather than treating the 'symptoms'.

Never make assumptions based on textbook theories around Autism either. This occurs far too frequently, particularly as parents who feel lost and helpless turn to the 'experts' for answers, only to be misdirected by the latest theory or piece of research surrounding a particular 'Autistic characteristic'.

Importantly, it's essential to rule out any possible organic cause for behavioural, diet and sleep issues before you start addressing

potential anxiety triggers or sensory responses. This is particularly true for the person who communicates in ways other than direct speech.

As parents, if we can put away the assumptions of incapacity about our children – because they are too young or because they are Autistic – and instead enable them in order to constructively empower their own natural communication and learning ability, we are far more likely to gain a better insight into what they are all about. Even if they cannot tell us directly.

This means recognising that our job as a parent is to interpret our children's own unique language – the one hardwired into their DNA - and that they are our teachers to the same extent as we are theirs.

When behaviours speak volumes
One of the more common (and I believe damaging) Autistic stigmas, particularly in those cases classified by the medical fraternity as 'severe' or 'extreme', is to do with "self injurious behaviours" or SIB.

This term used to describe actions like 'head banging' or biting oneself, leads parents to assume that their child is purposefully injuring him or herself and in turn, makes us feel like a helpless onlooker. It immediately engenders a sense of fear and defeat in mums and dads, who are left questioning and wondering:

- Is he seeking sensory input?
- Is he experiencing sensory overload from lights or sounds?
- Is something causing him physical distress?

The bottom line is, we are often left questioning and consulting endless experts and internet sites that all profess different theories and in turn, we become ever more panicked about finding some way to prevent our child from harming themselves.

But what if the so-called self-injurious behaviour was entirely out of your child's control? What if it was not simply the manifestation of a behaviour, but a symptom of some underlying issue; an issue the person is trying desperately to communicate, in a world that hinges on such a tiny window of acknowledged interaction, i.e. verbal exchange?

When most people get angry or emotional or have some kind of physical pain, they can scream, yell or talk about whatever is bothering them and release their anxiety or frustration in what our world considers more 'acceptable' ways.

But this isn't necessarily the case for everyone. Some of us express our pain or fear or anxiety in a different way. Moreover, many Autistic children who are said to exhibit SIB have incredibly high tolerance to physical pain. They still feel pain, but their brain interprets the sensation in a different way.

Then there are numerous documented instances, such as one from Autistic mother, advocate and author Judy Endow, around organic issues that are overlooked due to the behaviours being dismissed as self-injurious or, worse still, purposeful attempts to gain attention and be willfully defiant.

On her blog, Judy writes of an episode where a little girl banged her head into walls several times a day and had actually given herself a concussion. When this behaviour was observed for a period of time, it was assumed the girl head banged whenever she was asked to do something she did not wish to do.

A behaviour shaping and reward system was implemented in light of this theory, however when it proved ineffective after 6 months, further investigations were conducted. It was subsequently discovered that the little girl had a severe case of head lice which when treated, eradicated the head banging completely.

In another instance, Judy explains how a little boy with proprioceptive issues was assumed to be "pitching a fit" because he would drop to the floor yelling, "No, no no!" when walking through the door of his classroom.

In actuality, when he walked through the doorway with other children, the excessive movement along with spatial and lighting changes caused his sense of proprioception to 'bottom out'.

All it took to help this little boy was allowing him to leave the classroom with just one other person – preferably an adult who could hold his hand and alleviate some of the proprioception issues he was experiencing.

Judy says assumptions made around incapacity or wilfulness, aligned with certain individual behaviours, cause us to "assign negative character traits to our children". In turn, we can fail to notice the real underlying problems these children are trying to communicate and worse still, take away a little bit of their humanity.

> When today's brain scientists talk Asperger's, there's no mention of damage—just difference. Neurologists have not identified anything that's missing or ruined in the Asperger brain. That's a very important fact. We are not like the unfortunate people who've lost millions of neurons through strokes, drinking, lead poisoning, or accidental injury. Our brains are complete; it's just the interconnections that are different.

JOHN ELDER ROBISON

16. MAKING ALLOWANCES FOR AUTISM IN YOUR LIFE

When you accept your Autistic child, you will better understand how their different way of processing the world impacts their life on a daily basis. Sensory issues are an excellent and obvious example.

Think about grocery shopping. I'm sure some of you are having flashbacks to a failed supermarket outing in the not too distant past. But rather than recalling that experience with fear and frustration at how it all went 'terribly wrong', think for a moment about how much expectation was built around that shopping trip.

Of course in the first instance, you expect that you can take your child to the grocery store and they will behave impeccably. Then there's the judgment from onlookers that this is a child having a tantrum and the expectation that you, as their parent, should be able to "control them".

But stop for a minute and think empathetically about your Autistic child's experience of a trip to the grocery store, minus the expectation of how that experience 'should' look.

It's an endless assault on their senses, with fluorescent lights, elevator music and constant visual stimulation in row upon row of brightly coloured packaging. Not to mention the din from all those rusted shopping trolley wheels and beeping registers.

Anxiety and/or excitement invariably takes hold, triggering the brain's chemical receptors to warn us this is time for fight or flight and, well, one or both happen right there and then.

I remember walking into a very large undercover shopping centre one Christmas many years ago. It was a notoriously busy place at the best of times, so why I decided to try my luck during the festive season I have no idea.

After cutting laps of the carpark for almost an hour, I found a space and silently congratulated myself for remaining relatively calm. However, as soon as I walked into the climate-controlled mecca of retail worship, I was assaulted from all angles!

I turned around and walked straight back out and have never returned to this day. I now maintain at least a 50-yard perimeter between shops and myself in the 48 hour lead up to Christmas if I can help it!

In that instance, I had the ability to turn around and leave. I was not compelled to stay in that space, which I could not possibly tolerate, by anyone else.

My point is, by accepting your child's Autism; you are more likely to work with it rather than against it, in the sense that you expect them to 'behave normally' in various social settings.

Do you have to take your Autistic child to the shops for a marathon retail expedition? Because I can guarantee that after the first hour, you'll be regretting doing so!

I'm not suggesting that you can never take your Autistic child into that sort of environment. But you need to be prepared, you need to help them to prepare and you need to slowly desensitise them to the chaos of experience.

I've spoken to parents who have literally spent the first dozen trips to the shops just trying to get their children past the automatic doors without freaking out. When they succeed at this first effort, they slowly build up until they can manage an entire shopping trip with very little trauma. But it takes time and understanding.

Slowly, you will give your child the skills and confidence to self-soothe and self-manage in situations they might otherwise find too confronting to handle. In the meantime, you are the person they look to for security, for comfort and above all, for acceptance.

Subtle brain differences often cause people like me to respond differently—strangely even—to common life situations. Most of us have a hard time with social situations; some of us feel downright crippled. We get frustrated because we're so good at some things, while being completely inept at others. There's just no balance. It's a very difficult way to live, because our strengths seem to contrast so sharply with our weaknesses. "You read so well, and you're so smart! I can't believe you can't do what I told you. You must be faking!" I heard that a lot as a kid.

JOHN ELDER ROBISON

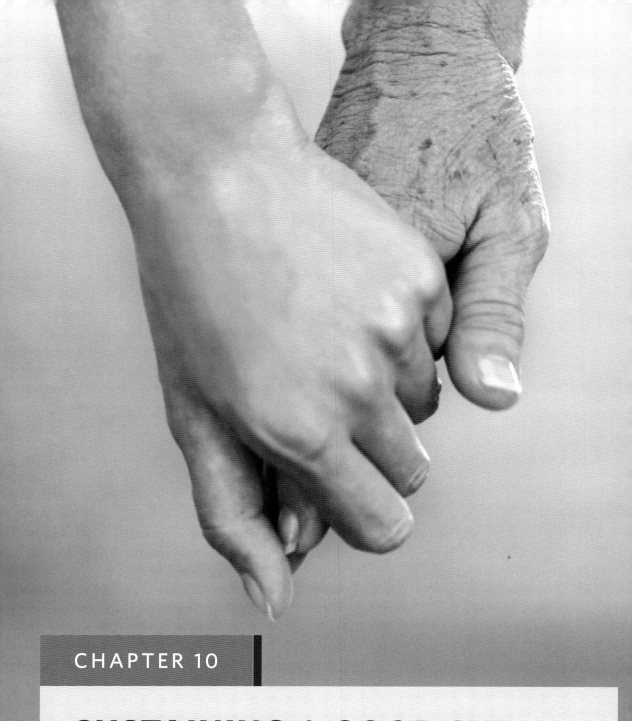

CHAPTER 10

SUSTAINING A GOOD SUPPORT NETWORK

Accepting an Autism diagnosis is much easier when you have a good support network around you, particularly people who understand the Autistic experience firsthand.

The risk of isolation when dealing with a difference as misunderstood as Autism is very real. And given the everyday challenges that can quickly overwhelm parents, who are often sleep deprived and confused as to how to respond to various behaviours and anxiety triggers, many families can find themselves in a type of self-imposed home detention.

One of the first things you need to let go of as an Autism parent is the fear of being judged. I recall a number of shopping trips that ended with our daughter having a complete sensory meltdown, as I fled the disapproving glares of onlookers feeling injured or close to tears, or both at the same time.

I wanted to scream at these strangers for making me feel inadequate as a parent. What gave them the right to shake their heads disparagingly and make assumptions about my child and my ability to 'control' her?

The answer is nothing. Autism might come with numerous challenges, but one of the most precious gifts it endows us with is empathy. It teaches us tolerance and makes us perceive the world very differently.

As an Autism parent, I look at other mums and dads as comrades, just trying to navigate a hyper-sensorial, confronting world with children who struggle to make sense of the assault on their little bodies and developing minds.

I don't really know why parents are not more supportive of one another. We can't possibly understand what is happening in anyone else's life, what challenges they might have experienced just to make it out the door dressed that day.

When we recognise that we are all just doing the best we can with the hand we have been dealt, it makes judgment empty and meaningless. It makes the misguided stares and silent critics insignificant.

Why do people feel compelled to judge one another? Because we are fractured and fragmented, all scattered on different winds. And we are taught that to survive, it's every man, woman and child for him or herself.

We are conditioned from a very young age to believe that we have to win, no matter what it takes or how it might disconnect us from our fellow human beings.

Therein lies the need for us to speculate about the shortcomings of others. We look at them as the enemy, whose weaknesses we need to count in order to take them on. We want to believe they are as powerless as we feel, so we tear them down with negative assumptions.

If we would just decide to be kind, caring, compassionate and connected, the need for such thinking would be eradicated. We would think only of ways to benefit the human collective of which we are a part, making it better for all.

17. AVOIDING FAMILY AND SOCIAL ISOLATION

Unfortunately there will be those in your family and friendship circles, who simply won't 'get it'. Some might try really hard to understand, some might nod politely and tune out when you start 'talking Autism' and then there are those who will insist there is 'nothing wrong' with your child! They just need a "firm hand"…essentially 'better parenting' is the unspoken implication.

You can do one of three things when confronted with this type of attitude:

1. Accept they think that way for their own reasons and just move right along with life.
2. Talk to them; explain what Autism means in your world and how it makes your child different and therefore, their experience of the world around them different.
3. Stew on their words and question yourself senseless about all the things you are 'doing wrong' and how dismally you are failing as a parent.

In my experience, you'll do all of the above at various stages. Judgment is never easy to cop and how you respond is entirely dependent on the type of person you are. But the fact is, you need support in your life and even if those people within your circles don't get it, all they really need to do is accept.

Part of the process of acceptance is education and understanding. Rather than shunning friends and family in fear of judgment, invite them into your world so they can see the Autistic experience firsthand. Explain the Autistic perspective and importantly, let them grow to know your child and the unique being they are by developing their own relationship with them.

This is where advocacy truly starts for Autism parents – in the home. It's our attitude and preparedness to allow our child to be the person they are, that influences how others will perceive and respond to them.

So be patient and be persistent. It just might pay off when it comes to maintaining your familial bonds and sustaining important support networks. Family can be problematic at times, but they can also be an unconditional blessing.

So what about the practicalities? How do you prevent family and social isolation…or more importantly, how do you strike a balance between the time you need for yourself and your family, and the time you need to extend your scope of interaction with the big wide world?

Here are a few tips that might help to get you thinking of ways to gain some harmony between the Autistic journey and your friends and family…

1. Don't make everything about Autism!

The temptation to talk to everyone about 'the Autism' will be very real. It becomes your life, as you scrutinise your child's every move trying to work out where 'the Autism' starts and finishes. Let me save you some time…don't bother!

Autism doesn't start or finish for your child – it's just who they are. Accept this and you'll save a lot of valuable hours looking for answers that your child gives you every moment of every day, just by being themselves.

Part of acceptance is allowing your child to simply be. So many struggles – physical, mental and emotional – stem from the frustration of Autistic children not being heard, or having their personalities smothered.

Sometimes it's nice to give your child room to just be who they are, without worrying about how the label defines them to us, or to Aunty Jean.

2. Embrace your child's quirks and the differences they bring to your world. When you do so, others will follow suit and acceptance won't be too far behind. Acceptance goes a long way to having friends and family come to acknowledge that before them is a child, a person. We want people to see Aislinn - not Aislinn the Autistic child - but Aislinn.

3. Welcome difference into your inner circle. I'm not talking about a token Autistic friend! There are people with all sorts of quirks and differences floating through our lives at various junctures… well; a lot of them float through my world – but then like attracts like!

Acknowledge and celebrate difference within your networks, not as a deficiency of character, but as a strength. At the same time, speak of the challenges that can come from those differences in a world that celebrates 'same'. Doing so will make your bonds stronger and Autistic acceptance far more probable.

4. Communicate. It can be easy to isolate oneself when Autism enters our world. Finding rejection where we hoped for acceptance can cause us to shut off from those we feel are silently or openly judging us. At these times, it's important to express how you feel if possible.

I know that I am alive; I breathe, move, talk and function just like any other Human Being. However, I understand (because it has been said to me) that other people perceive me as being different to them. My difference expresses itself in various ways, (egocentricity, eccentricity, and emotional immaturity) but, in particular, in my uneven skill ability.

Life seems to me to be like a video that I can watch, but not partake in. I sense that I live my life 'Behind Glass'. However, at times I am completely taken up with an obsession or a perception that may dominate my existence and make it easy to stay focused. For me, such times mean that I feel 'connected' to life. Life, for me, takes on meaning and purpose.

JOHN ELDER ROBISON

Sometimes you may not be able to articulate your feelings in the moment, and that's okay. Just take some time to process your emotions and importantly, digest that information for your own self-reflection.

But it's good to let people know which comments and suggestions are welcome as genuine offerings of assistance, and which ones are not at all helpful. Remember, experiences are very personal things – based on our own unique perception of people or circumstances we encounter on our journey.

We might be looking at the same thing, but each seeing something entirely different.

18. MAINTAINING YOUR NETWORKS & BUILDING NEW ONES

How you handle the initial Autism diagnosis will speak volumes to your child and those in your familial and friendship networks, about who they are and how you feel about their difference.

Remember a diagnosis is merely confirmation in the form of a label as to whom you already knew your child to be – the word did not change them overnight. So it's important to talk to family and friends about the diagnosis as a matter of fact element in your already different world.

Acknowledge that others around you might have certain feelings about the diagnosis, due to common stereotypes and stigmas clouding their own misguided perceptions. And talk to them about the realities of your child's difference in this world and how it impacts their experience and expression.

Importantly, make allowances for your child when interacting with friends and family. Don't pressure them to 'perform' through on demand displays of affection and polite social mores.

The more you coerce them to give Great Aunt Gloria a kiss and say 'thank you', the more resistance and anxiety triggered behaviours you will likely end up dealing with each time Great Aunt Gloria pops over for a cup of tea!

One of the best things you can do is share information you're given during the assessment of your child from people like Occupational Therapists and Speech Therapists.

Being presented with official paperwork that outlines things like sensory issues or speech delays will potentially open up the channels of acceptance and understanding within your support network.

Forming new networks

While it's critical to keep the lines of communication open when it comes to your existing networks, take the opportunity to form new connections with others living the Autistic experience.

Never will you feel quite so understood and accepted as with other Autism parents. In most of the support groups I've encountered, judgment is left at the door, making way for empathy and knowing nods as mums and dads share their stories, along with large doses of caffeine!

These are people who live the experience every day. In these support groups parents come together to laugh, cry and most of all, learn a lot about themselves and the wonders of their respective Autistic journeys.

There is one disclaimer here though… I would caution parents to be careful of the group they end up in. While most are full of hope and reassurance, some can be incredibly negative toward Autism.

I get it. We are often left to cope alone and can therefore become easily overwhelmed, seeing Autism as the cause of all our perceived 'problems'.

But while it's nice to be able to vent occasionally about a world that fails to understand your child and your family's experience, these support groups should be about lifting one another up and showing a unique solidarity and connection. They should also be about acceptance!

19. WHY SUPPORT IS ESSENTIAL

It all comes back to that need for connection I've been talking about, a need for love and understanding. It's nice to think we have those friends and family members who are not going to condemn us for having an untidy house, because they 'get' that we've had three years of broken sleep.

Genuine human connection, filled with empathy, acceptance and understanding, is just as important to our survival as the air we breathe, the water we drink and the food we consume.

Without it, we are starved of affection and affiliation with our fellow human beings and we feel adrift in the world.

This in turn leads to depression and a general inability to cope with the daily pressures and demands of our modern life. Moreover, when we feel supported in ourselves, we are better able to support those around us.

> I've learned that every human being, with or without disabilities, needs to strive to do their best, and by striving for happiness you will arrive at happiness. For us, you see, having Autism is normal—so we can't know for sure what your 'normal' is even like. But so long as we can learn to love ourselves, I'm not sure how much it matters whether we're normal or Autistic.

NAOKI HIGASHIDA,
AUTHOR OF *THE REASON I JUMP*

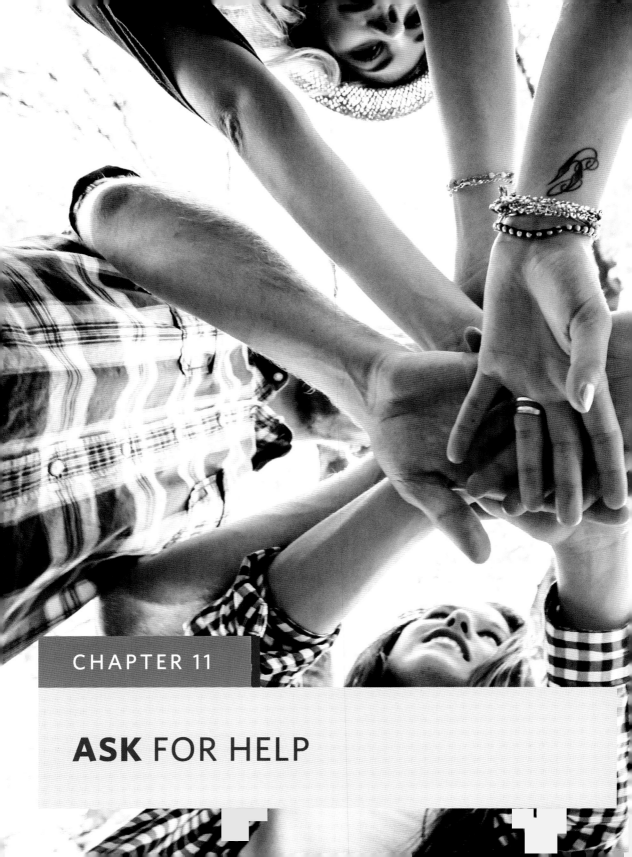

CHAPTER 11

ASK FOR HELP

How hard is it to ask for help these days? I detest having to ask for help, because it generally means traversing into systems and places that you really just don't want to have to go.

Usually these forays come with a lot of red tape and bureaucratic box ticking that leaves parents and carers, not to mention the adult Aspergian with a few executive functioning differences, feeling completely defeated.

At least this was my experience when the pre-school Aislinn was enrolling in suggested we apply for funding to secure an aide, who could assist with her transition.

The main requirement was an essay on my daughter's shortcomings, preferably penned or at least guided by me and focusing entirely on her "worst case scenario" moments. At no stage was I to mention anything positive, on that point they were quite insistent.

Essentially, the only thing that would attract money to my daughter's cause was a portrait of an aggressive, confrontational and disobedient little girl, with a series of extreme behavioural issues.

While getting to know Aislinn has not been an altogether constant or smooth path (getting to know another so intimately as you do your child never is really), we like to acknowledge those moments when she grows into herself a bit more, and in turn learns how to make the most of her difference in this world.

So yes, while this amazing little being definitely has her 'less than pleasant moments' with us, and us with her, as

all human beings have a tendency to do because of our inherent differences and similarities, there are far more wonderful times to cherish.

She is an amazing person who forever keeps you guessing. With her multi-dimensional personality and colourful personas, Aislinn has a presence, drive, determination and confidence that I wish I possessed half of when growing up.

But the fact is, when you're asking for help through official channels, they don't want to know about any of that. You have to be the 'squeaky wheel' and for some, asking for help is tantamount to admitting defeat; on a personal level, we think we have somehow failed as parents if we need assistance in life.

Many are reluctant to ask friends or family for help for various reasons – whether it be a fear of judgment over "not being able to cope", or just a sense that the people you would normally ask seem so busy with their own lives, you don't want to bother them.

The problem is, we are all meant to be helping one another through life in meaningful, connected ways. Not as 'social security' numbers talking to worker drones on the other end of a phone line, which is essentially what our cries for help have been reduced to.

Don't believe me? Call a government department looking for help and the first thing you'll be asked to provide, even before your name, is a social security or reference number – usually to a machine.

So yes, there will be times when you feel you desperately need some help, guidance, direction or just a willing ear. It's a natural human need to share our burdens with others and find empathy and connection on all levels.

I guess what I'm trying to suggest is that to need help is human. To know what help you need and how to get it is smart. To understand that the help will often come with conditions that may not be entirely palatable, is very wise indeed…and will save you a lot of heartache.

I often tell people who are putting on the advocate hat for their child, to assume a role of logic and reasoning. Try to make the process as systematic for you, as it is for the systems you're working in, as difficult as that might seem.

If you can manage to do so, you will not only find it easier to rationalise the awful hoops you'll be asked to jump through in order to finally get what you require. You'll also be one step ahead when it comes to working your way through their processes and procedures.

Importantly, expect no help at all. I know it sounds strange to suggest that you ask for help, all the while expecting none to be forthcoming. But the fact is, if you get your hopes up about some level of assistance that you're pinning any chance of success on, you could end up bitterly disappointed and are more likely to lose sight of other alternatives that might be available.

20. KNOWING WHAT YOU NEED AND WHEN YOU NEED IT.

Sometimes all you need is a willing ear, or a shoulder to lean on when you're completely exhausted and ready to drop. At other times, you might need a more literal financial, physical or emotional crutch, and that's perfectly okay.

The key for parents is to not ignore or push aside your own needs, while trying to help your child or children. This can be difficult, as our maternal and paternal drive to provide and nurture can become overwhelming. This is particularly true of many 'special needs' parents I know.

We can be like mama and papa bears fiercely protecting our cubs! But I have seen the consequences of being unwilling to acknowledge the need to seek or ask for help, which can be devastating to relationships and for mental and physical health and wellbeing.

As mentioned above, if you can identify your needs – and this in itself is a process of trying to work through your situation with calm, rational logic – then you're one step closer to addressing any issues you might be experiencing effectively.

The key is to take action before you become overwhelmed with the problem at hand, because when you get caught up in crisis mode, it's difficult to accurately assess and acknowledge your true needs.

You know best

Often, we are told what our children need by the 'experts' who diagnose them. They require this amount of therapy, with this specialist, this often.

Feeling besieged by information overload and fear as to what the consequences might be if they don't get immediate help with their child, many parents panic and start ferrying their child from one appointment to another and another.

Often, necessary and rigorous processes to measure outcomes and effectiveness of therapy(s) are not adequately established, such as a comprehensive therapy diary, or regular meetings between all therapists involved with the child to discuss progress.

I believe that more practitioners should educate their patients (or parents of children they have as clients) around becoming partners in the therapeutic process; not to be told what to do, with an expectation that you'll blindly obey, but as someone who is their own best expert to be consulted on a level playing field.

Before you allow professionals (who see you for all of half an hour every month or so) to determine your needs or those of your child, make yourself an important part of the process.

What I mean by that is, be confident in your knowledge of your child and family and use that confidence to have a clear voice and be the owner and leader of your Autism journey.

Establish a relationship with those from whom you seek guidance and assistance and direct these relationships to derive maximum benefit and the best possible outcomes for your situation, whatever they might be.

I've said on many occasions, Autism requires so much more than a 'one size fits all' response, and everyone's needs throughout the journey are vastly different.

What do you need?

One of the best ways to establish your needs is to first be clear about your goals and where you would like to be as your journey progresses. Write down your desired outcomes and importantly, make them measurable and make all those involved in the process accountable.

For instance, your goal might be to manage a half hour shopping trip minus any incident you couldn't overcome without completely losing the plot. We've all been there – shops can be Hell!

Within this goal, set clear parameters around what you want to achieve and how that success will look for you. Give your goals clarity and meaning in your reality, by attaching them to your physical surroundings.

This could be as literal as noting them down – as words or images – and then sticking them up in prominent places throughout your home, where you will be reminded of what all your hard work is heading towards, every day.

It does not matter what sixty-six percent of people do in any particular situation. All that matters is what you do.

JOHN ELDER ROBISON,
AUTHOR OF *LOOK ME IN THE EYE*

Don't get diverted

Distractions are everywhere when you parent a 'special needs' child. You have so much misinformation to contend with on a daily basis, often coming from a trusted source, which makes it even more difficult to see the wood for the trees.

People will suggest all kinds of things that you really should try. This is where it comes in handy to be a fact seeker. If you love learning new things, then you'll appreciate the Autistic journey. If it's anything at all, it's definitely a steep learning curve around what you thought you knew about life!

Educating yourself by truly validating your child as the individual they are, not the label they are assigned, is essential in this space so that you are less likely to become a statistic. Not a statistic of Autism, but of broader society's complete misunderstanding of the true neuro-divergent/Autistic experience.

You risk robbing your experience as a parent with your children in those first precious years, if you place too much faith in what medical professionals tell you about your son or daughter.

Remember – they do not know your little people! They see them for such minimal periods of time – the blink of an eye – and usually when they're at their most anxious. They see them in isolation of the Autism deficiency model.

The same goes for teaching and school staff, who admittedly spend far more time with your offspring in the classroom than their doctors ever will. But who also experience your children at their most anxious and sensory overwhelmed.

The point is you know your child best, so you need to maintain control when it comes to how they experience their own Autistic journey. You can help to determine a far more positive life experience by being invested and getting to know their needs and your own.

21. LEARNING WHEN AND HOW TO SAY "NO" AS WELL AS "YES"

Many of us feel compelled to say yes to everything, lest we offend someone or let him or her down. In a world where we are encouraged to expect something always, this can be a very real concern.

I know I've had alleged friendships that hinged entirely on me being readily available for a lengthy phone conversation when the other person just felt the need to vent at someone.

But when you realise that time spent with your children is far more valuable than these 'go nowhere' relationships, it becomes easier to challenge those things that drain your energy needlessly, and eventually bid them farewell.

Often time will reveal relationships that are healthy in your world with Autism, as opposed to those that are toxic and best left to die a natural death. But in the meantime, it's helpful to recognise those who enrich your life with their presence and those whose absence would make your world a better place.

When you are focused on your goals and needs and those of your family, you will be more likely to have the confidence and conviction to accept experiences that will get you one step closer to reaching your ideal objectives, while side stepping the things that will get in the way and trip you up.

Why was it considered normal for a girl to live for fashion and makeup, but not car engines or bugs? And what about sports fanatics? My mum had a boy-friend who would flip out if he missed even a minute of a football game. Wouldn't that be what doctors considered Autistic behaviour?

TARA KELLY, *HARMONIC FEEDBACK*

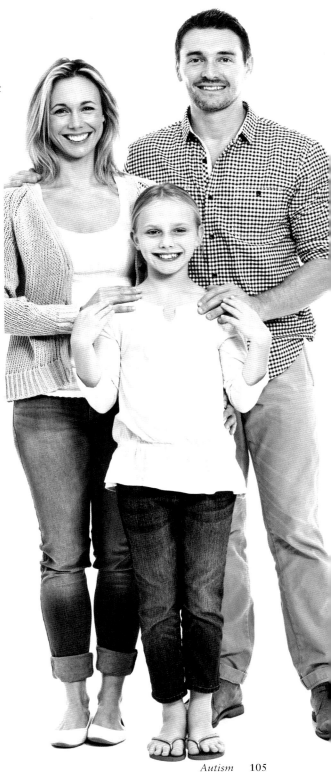

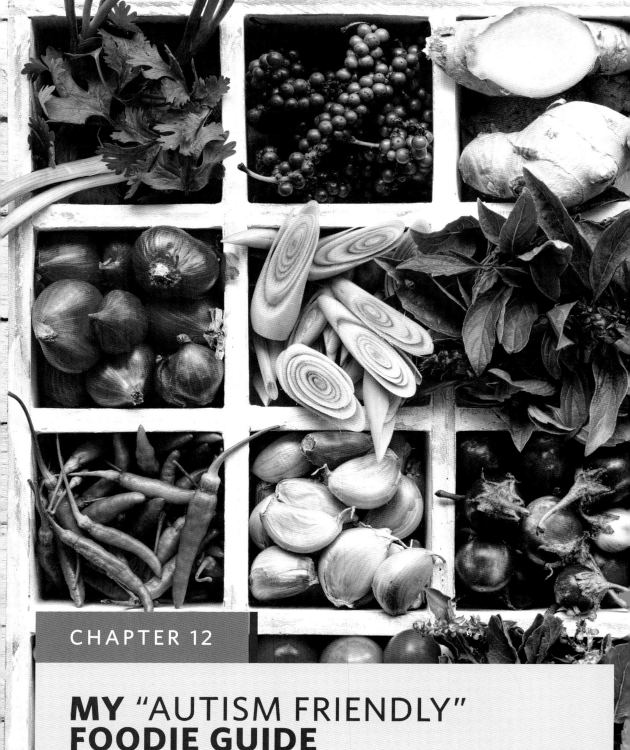

CHAPTER 12

MY "AUTISM FRIENDLY"
FOODIE GUIDE

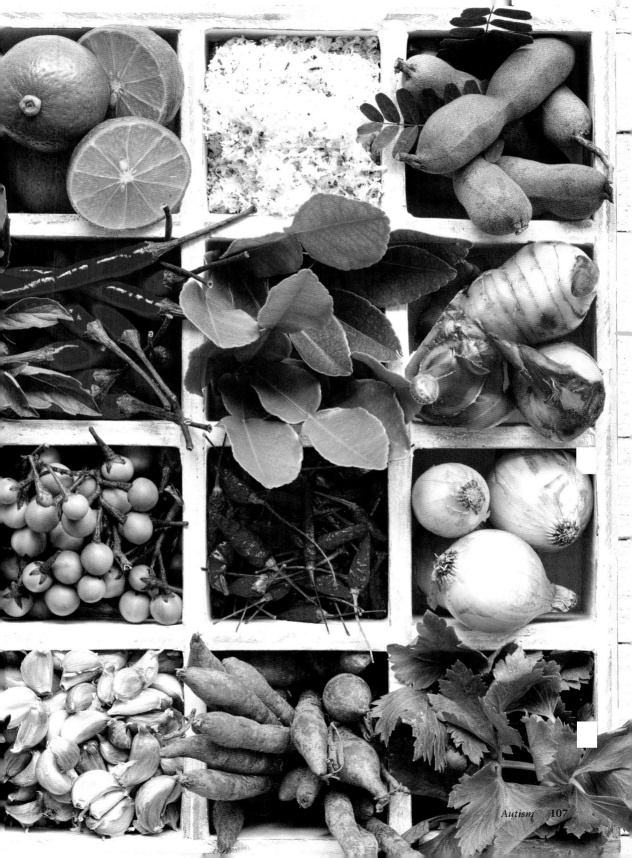

Fussy eating generally goes hand in hand with Autism. Whether it be for sensory reasons, a reluctance to step out of one's comfort zone and try new things, a physiological (organic) imbalance of some kind, or a combination of all the above, food intake restrictions are common among Aspergians and Autistics.

Some will only eat certain colours and textures; others refuse to try any new tastes beyond a limited repertoire of sweet, salty or sour.

For our family food is a very important aspect of how we live, not just the Autistic experience now, but the diabetic one too. As with everything else, we have thrown away the rulebook as to what constitutes a 'normal' diet.

Doing food differently these days entails cooking from scratch, eating organic and refusing to acknowledge anything that comes from a packet as having any nutritional value.

It's not an easy path to take in a world where processed foods have become 'normal' everyday fare. High sugar, high carb, high fat food in abundance is now the standardised western diet and if you don't succumb to this mentality, you're viewed as some type of monster who tortures your offspring with food deprivation of the cruellest kind.

The truth about food is this…we have been fed a big smorgasbord of lies for many years. The so-called 'Healthy Food Pyramid' we are taught about in school was developed to keep a then ailing agricultural industry afloat. It was devised for profit over the health of people.

We are the only mammals who consume the milk of other animals, we have been led to believe that sugary, processed junk is 'normal' and we are all suffering on many levels as a result.

Our digestive system and gut is like the control room of our entire existence. Not only does it keep us alive, it also controls our emotions and thoughts and in turn, our physicality and actions.

The food we put in our bodies influences and triggers intricate and complex chemical responses in our brain's hard wiring – releasing all sorts of hormones and even influencing the electrical impulses that determine the health of our mind's neural pathways.

There have been many studies around the link between certain mental health and developmental concerns – almost modern day conditions with the current prevalence of depression and anxiety – and the effects of diet and lifestyle.

I'm not one of those who suggest that diet 'causes' Autism. However, I absolutely believe in the power of food to heal all aspects of our body, including the many problematic co-morbidities that accompany Autism, such as anxiety and sensory processing issues.

That being said, and given that we have a strong genetic predisposition toward Celiac disease in our family, with Jason suffering from a complete gluten intolerance since the age of thirteen, Reilly's diagnosis was the final catalyst that coerced me into taking the foodie road less travelled and making our household gluten and dairy free.

Like I said, this path isn't as easy as relying on the 'golden arches' to deliver up some plastic fantastic concoction that we can convince ourselves is food because it's 'convenient'.

A foodie community

As with the Autism community, I've noticed that the 'healthy eating' movement is largely facilitated by a group of mums who, due to one health crisis or another within their family, have recognised the need to be, well…'different'.

It's these wonderful, creative types who have concocted some of my favourite recipes that I now rely on when I'm having one of 'those day's', where the kids refuse to try anything remotely new that doesn't involve their long time staple – yep, you guessed it, bread and dairy!

Thankfully we have never been a big junk food family, but overcoming the 'that's not what I normally eat' argument has been a struggle, I admit. I have sat at the dinner table, surveying three untouched meals and cried in defeat. I've ranted and raved and reasoned about how 'I'm doing this for your own good'. All the while knowing my words are falling on deaf ears!

Like I said, this is the path of most resistance, because it's the one less travelled. But the battle isn't only worth it for my children's health, it's completely necessary.

So I say a big thank you to the wonderful mums out there who are blazing healthy food trails all over the World Wide Web. Like the Autism community, there's a solidarity in healthy eating circles that I admire and respect – we all appreciate what it means to walk to the beat of a different drum.

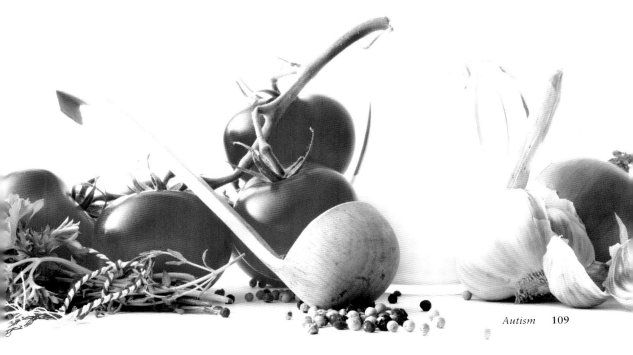

QUINOA BREAD WITH AVOCADO & POACHED EGG

This Quinoa bread recipe is by one of my favourite food bloggers, Australia's very own healthy chef, Teresa Cutter.

INGREDIENTS

300g (1 ³/₄ cups) whole uncooked quinoa seeds

60g (¹/₄ cup) whole chia seeds

250ml (1 cup) water

60ml (¹/₄ cup) olive oil

¹/₂ tsp bicarb soda

¹/₂ tsp sea salt

Juice from ¹/₂ lemon

METHOD

1. Preheat a fan forced oven to 160°C/320°F.

2. Soak the quinoa in plenty of cold water in the fridge overnight.

3. Soak the chia seeds in ¹/₂ cup (125ml) of the water until gel like – this can be done overnight as well, but just give it a few stirs at the beginning.

4. Drain the quinoa and rinse well, making sure all water is removed.

5. Place the quinoa in a food processor and add the chia gel, ¹/₂ cup (125ml) of water, olive oil, bicarb soda, sea salt and lemon juice.

6. Mix for 3 minutes until it resembles a batter consistency with some whole quinoa still left in the mix.

7. Spoon into a loaf tin lined with baking paper and bake for 1 ¹/₂ hours until firm to touch and it bounces back when pressed with your fingers.

8. Remove from the oven and cool for 30 minutes in the tin then remove from the tin and cool completely on a rack or board. The bread should be slightly moist in the middle and crisp on the outside. Cool completely before eating.

9. Top with a runny, poached free range egg and sliced avocado, season with salt and pepper to taste.

10. The bread can be wrapped and stored in the fridge for up to one week or frozen for up to 3 months.

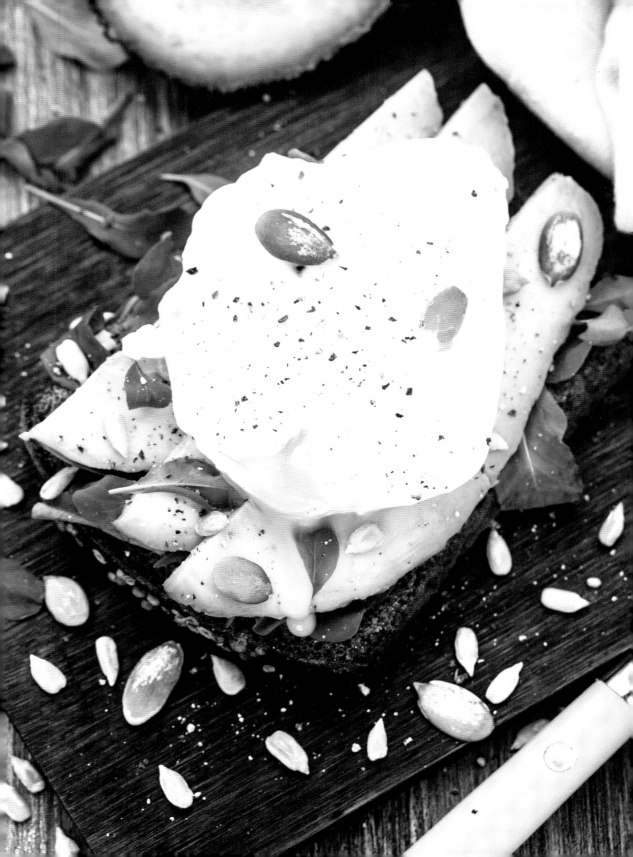

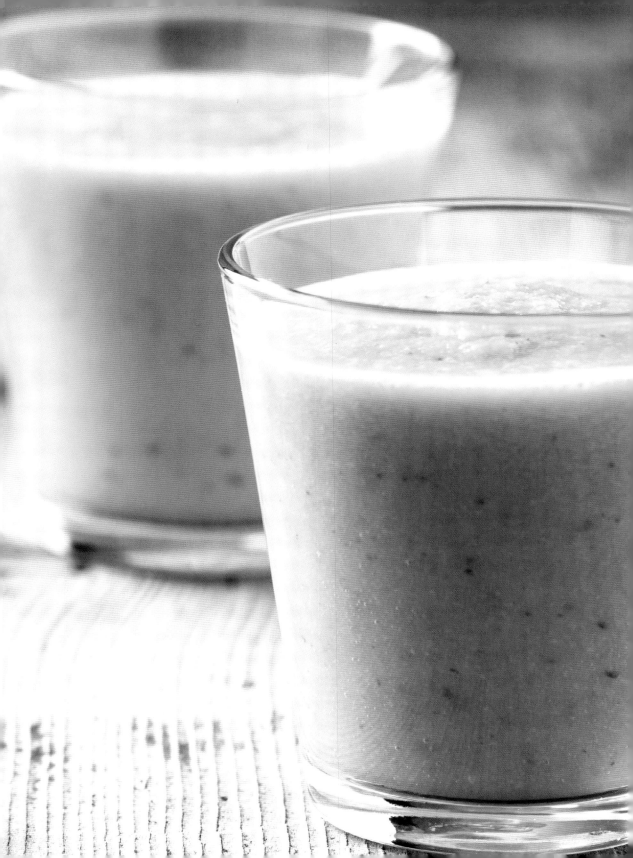

GREEN SMOOTHIE

INGREDIENTS

1 Granny Smith apple – peeled, cored and sliced

Handful of spinach or kale - washed

1 cup (125ml) coconut water

Ice

Flesh of 1 small avocado

Juice from $1/2$ lemon

Small nob of fresh ginger

METHOD

1. Blitz all ingredients in a high-speed blender until smooth. If you like a juice that's less fibrous, you might want to strain the mix through a fine sieve or nut milk bag.

2. Boost your juice with spirulina, wheat-grass, chlorophyll or aloe vera for gut healing and alkalising effects.

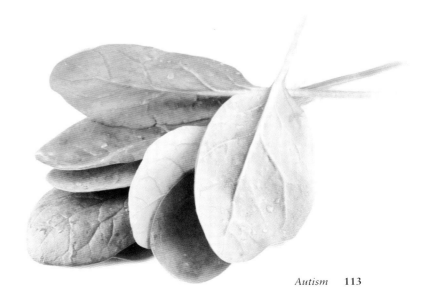

FISH & POTATO CAKES

INGREDIENTS

500g/1 lb potatoes

300g/10 oz white flesh fish
(fresh or frozen)

Olive oil

Salt and pepper

1 tbsp spelt flour

2 free range eggs

1 tbsp chopped chives

2 tbsp chopped parsley

2 cups (200g) quinoa flakes

Zest and juice of 1 lemon

METHOD

1. Peel and dice the potatoes, add to a pot of salted boiling water and bring to the boil.

2. Coat the fish generously in olive oil and salt and place in a steaming basket or colander.

3. When the potatoes are about half cooked, put the colander on top of the pot and continue cooking on medium heat for about 10 minutes.

4. Put the fish in a small bowl and use the same colander to drain the potatoes.

5. Return the potatoes to the pot and allow to sit for a few minutes then mash and let cool before placing in a large bowl.

6. Add the flour, egg, chopped herbs, $\frac{1}{2}$ cup (50g) quinoa flakes, lemon zest and juice and flake the fish into the bowl.

7. Mix and mash together the ingredients then season with a good pinch of salt and pepper.

8. Divide the mixture into 10-12 round fishcakes, about 2cm/1 inch thick.

9. Coat in the remaining quinoa flakes, place on baking paper and sit in the fridge to firm for 1 hour.

10. Coat the base of a frypan with about 1cm / $\frac{1}{2}$ inch deep of oil – canola, vegetable or grapeseed – and shallow fry the fish cakes on medium heat until they're golden, turning half way through cooking.

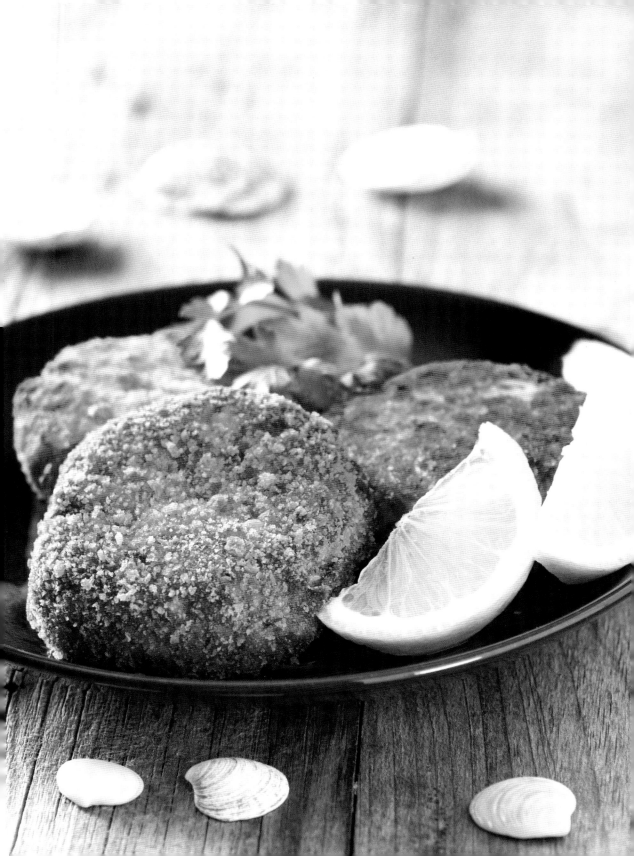

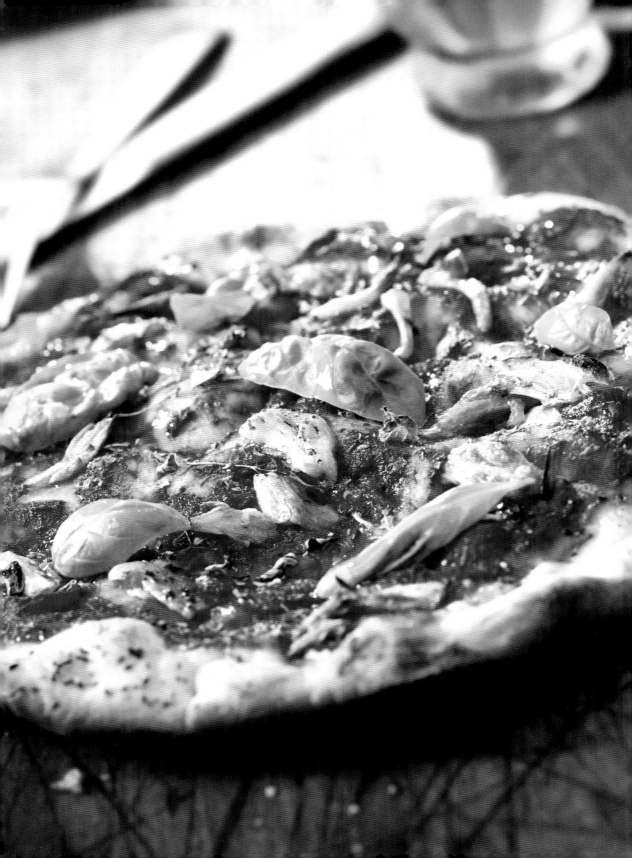

EASY PEAZY GLUTEN FREE PIZZA

INGREDIENTS

Pizza Base

1 cup (120g) gluten free self raising flour

1 cup (285g) Greek yoghurt (pot set preferred)

Tomato sauce

$1/2$ cup (125ml) tomato paste

1 tbsp sugar free tomato sauce

1 tbsp Worcestershire sauce (GF)

2 cloves minced or chopped garlic

Mixed Italian herbs

Salt & pepper to taste

METHOD

1. Combine the flour and yoghurt and mix into a dough. You may need to adjust the flour and yoghurt measures to ensure the dough the isn't too sticky.

2. Place a sheet of baking paper on the bench, dust lightly with more of the gluten free flour, turn out the dough and knead well for around 5-8 minutes. Dust your hands with flour to make kneading easier if required.

3. Shape the dough into a ball, cover with another sheet of baking paper and roll into a large circle of 1cm / $1/2$ inch thickness, or thicker depending on how you like your crust!

4. To make the tomato sauce, combine the tomato paste, tomato sauce, Worcestershire sauce, garlic, mixed Italian herbs and salt and pepper to taste.

5. Assemble the pizza with selected ingredients after topping with sauce, then place in a preheated oven at 180°C/350°F and cook until the cheese has melted and the crust is golden brown. Cooking times will vary depending on your oven, so check the pizza from around the 20 minute mark.

MINCE MAGIC MEATLOAF

INGREDIENTS

500g /1 lb quality minced beef

1 cup (150g) grated sweet potato

½ cup (70g) grated zucchini

½ cup (70g) grated carrot

3 cloves crushed garlic

1 finely diced brown onion

2 x 400g/14 oz tins crushed tomato or ½ bottle Passata sauce

2 tbsp tomato paste

1 tbsp tomato sauce

1 tbsp soy sauce

1 tbsp Worcestershire sauce

1 tsp turmeric

1 tsp mixed Italian herbs

1 free range egg

3 tbsp quinoa flakes

Salt and pepper to taste

Cheese for topping (optional)

METHOD

1. Preheat the oven to 180°C/350°F and line an oven tray with baking paper.

2. Combine all ingredients in a large bowl and mix together with your hands.

3. Shape into single serve mini-loafs and place on the oven tray.

4. Bake for 45 minutes, remove from the oven and sprinkle lightly with grated cheese (optional). Return the tray to the oven until the cheese melts and turns golden (approx 5 more minutes).

5. If baking without cheese, leave in the oven for 50 minutes before removing.

6. Serve with cauliflower or potato mash and seasonal steamed greens.

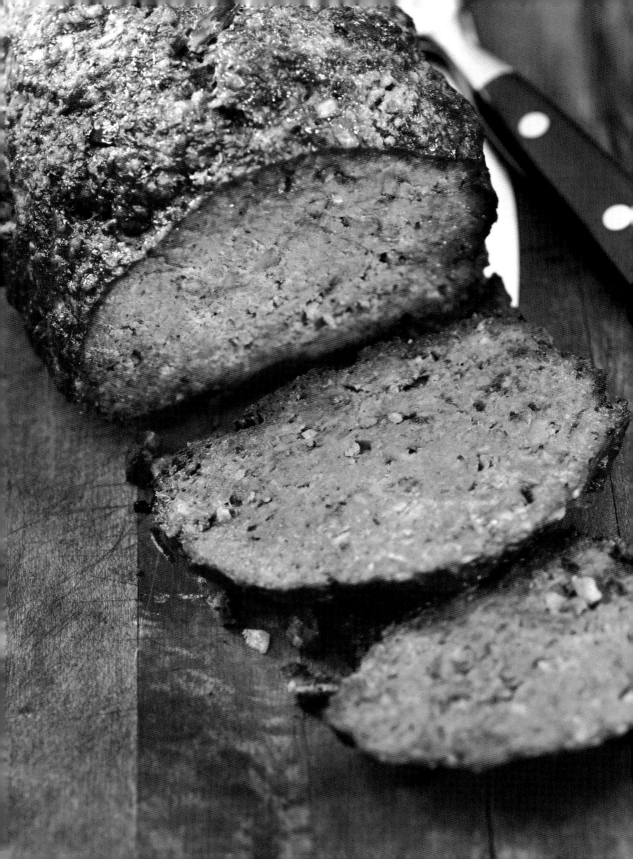

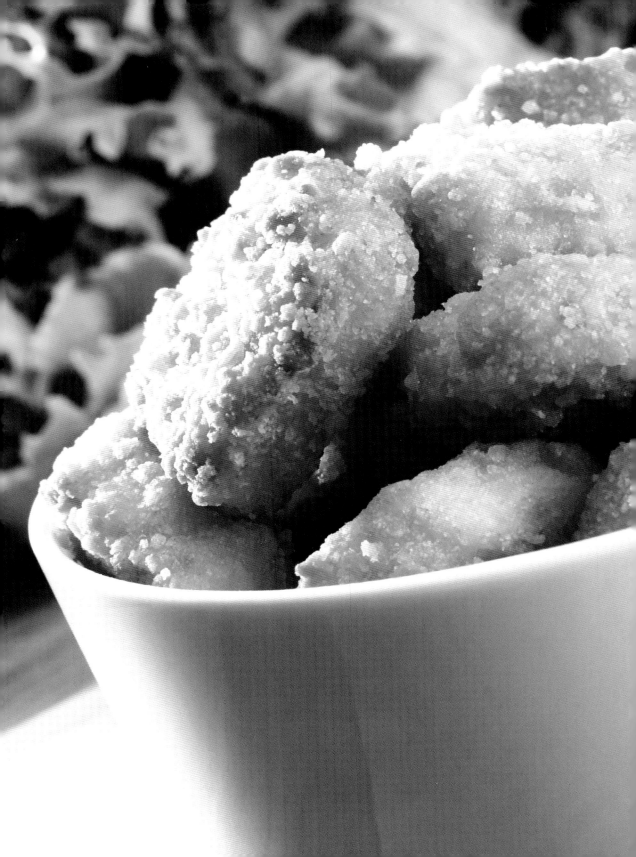

GLUTEN FREE CHICKEN NUGGETS

INGREDIENTS

3 free range eggs

1 tbsp Dijon mustard

1/4 cup (30g) gluten free all purpose flour

500g/1 lb chicken breast fillets

2 cups (500ml) good quality oil (coconut or rice bran oil)

Crumbing mix

1 cup (70g) gluten and sugar free cornflakes

1 cup (100g) quinoa flakes

2 cups (115g) gluten free rice crumbs (or crumbs made with stale gluten free bread)

1 cup (90g) parmesan cheese

1 tsp turmeric

Salt & pepper to taste

METHOD

1. Crush the cornflakes by placing them in a plastic bag, sealing without any air and bashing with a rolling pin or meat mallet.

2. Mix all the crumbing ingredients together in a large dish and season to taste.

3. In another dish, lightly beat the egg and Dijon mustard together.

4. Sprinkle the flour on a plate.

5. Slice the chicken breast fillets into nugget sized pieces (not too thick).

6. Coat each piece of chicken in flour, then dip in the egg/mustard wash and finally coat generously with the crumbing mix.

7. Heat enough oil for shallow frying in a large, deep pan.

8. Fry the chicken nuggets in batches, turning halfway through cooking to ensure both sides are golden brown.

QUINOA 'FRIED RICE'

INGREDIENTS

1 cup (180g) quinoa

2 tbsp olive oil

2 cloves minced garlic

1 brown onion or 1 small bunch of spring onions (finely diced)

2 free range eggs (lightly beaten)

$1/2$ cup (65g) baby corn

$1/2$ cup (65g) frozen peas

1 cup (150g) small broccoli florets

$1/2$ cup (70g) sliced zucchini

$1/2$ cup (70g) snow peas

Sauce

$1/4$ cup (60ml) soy sauce

2 tbsp sweet chilli sauce

1 tbsp honey

Salt and pepper to taste

METHOD

1. Soak, drain and cook the quinoa according to package instructions.

2. In a large wok or frying pan heat the olive oil, then add minced garlic and diced onion and fry off until transparent.

3. Add the vegetables and toss to cook, retaining their crispness.

4. Push the vegetables to one side and pour the egg into the pan.

5. Stir the egg to the consistency of a scramble, then mix through with the vegetables.

6. Reduce the heat and add the cooked quinoa to the pan, mix well.

7. To make the sauce combine the soy sauce, sweet chilli sauce, honey and salt and pepper to taste. Add the sauce to the quinoa rice and stir through before serving.

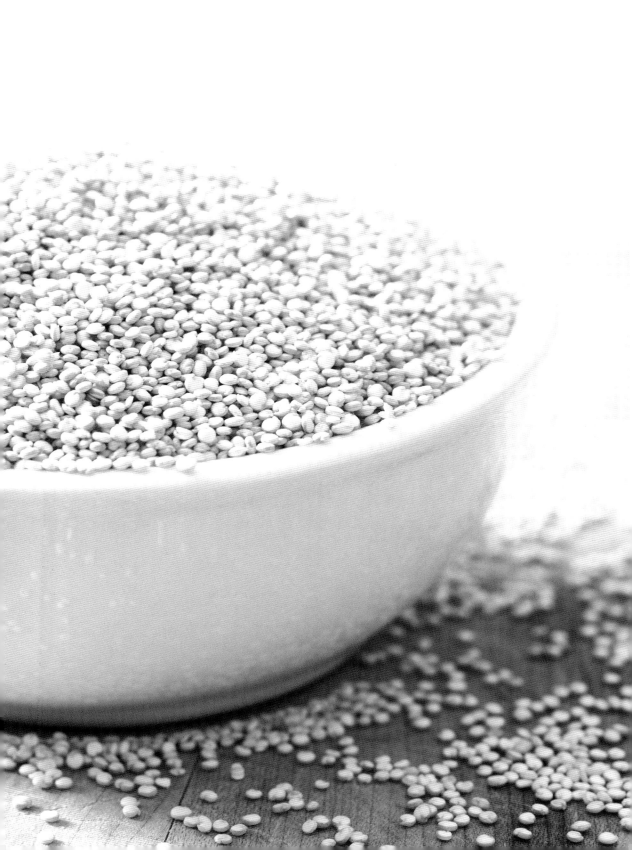

HOMEMADE HUMMUS DIP

INGREDIENTS

600g /1.3 lb canned chickpeas, drained and rinsed

3 garlic cloves, crushed

100ml (1/3 cup) olive oil

2 tbsp tahini paste

1 tsp ground cumin

Juice of 1 lemon

$1/4$ cup (60ml) water

Toasted Turkish bread, to serve

METHOD

1. Place the chickpeas, garlic, olive oil, tahini paste, cumin and lemon juice in a food processor and process until combined.

2. Add $1/4$ cup (60ml) of water and process again until smooth.

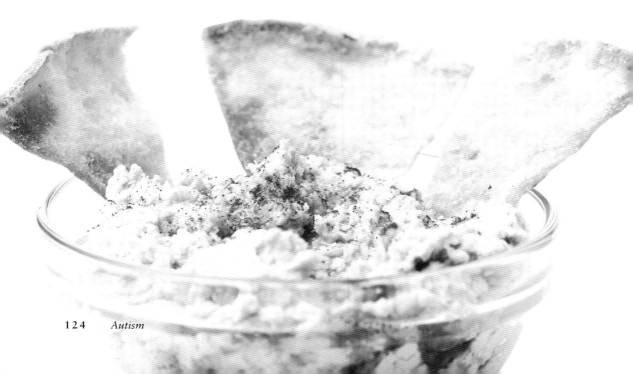

MOCK CHOC BARS

INGREDIENTS

First ingredients

1 cup (240g) almond butter

1/4 cup (60ml) plus 1 tbsp water

2 tbsp honey

1 tsp vanilla extract

1/8 tsp Stevia

1/2 cup (40g) shredded coconut

Second ingredients

1/2 cup (55g) organic raisins

1 tbsp chia seeds

1 tbsp flax meal

2 tsp cinnamon

1/4 tsp all spice

1/2 tsp baking powder

1/4 tsp salt

1/4 tsp baking soda

METHOD

1. Combine the first ingredients listed in a bowl and mix on low speed with an electric beater.

2. Add the second lot of ingredients and mix on low speed until combined.

3. Transfer the batter to a square or rectangular baking dish and spread evenly.

4. Bake at 170°C/340°F for around 25 minutes.

5. The slice is ready when a skewer comes out clean.

6. Allow to cool on the bench and refrigerate before slicing.

7. Keep in the fridge for up to a week.

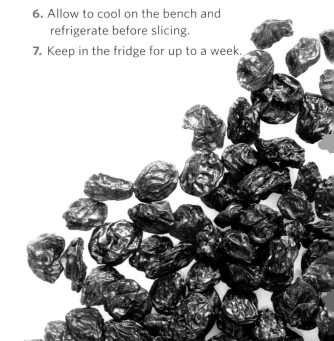

KALE CHIPS

INGREDIENTS

1 bunch fresh kale

dash of olive oil

dash of red wine vinegar

good pinch of Celtic sea salt or pink Himalayan salt crystals

METHOD

1. Pre-heat the oven to 150°C/300°F.
2. Wash and dry the kale thoroughly.
3. Strip the leaves from the stem (discard the stem as it can be very chewy) and tear into large, chip size pieces.
4. Place the kale in a bowl with olive oil, vinegar and salt and gently massage the leaves, coating thoroughly with the oil mixture.
5. Place the leaves on oven trays covered with baking paper in a single layer.
6. Bake for 10 minutes then rotate the trays and bake for a further 15 minutes, or until crisp.
7. Keep an eye on your chips as they can scorch easily.

GARLIC ROASTED BEANS

INGREDIENTS

2 cups (300g) organic green beans

olive oil

juice from ½ lemon

2 cloves minced garlic

Salt & pepper to taste

METHOD

1. Wash, top and tail the beans.
2. Preheat the oven to 175°C/350°F.
3. In a bowl, combine the olive oil, lemon juice and the garlic.
4. Toss the beans through the oil mixture.
5. Place the beans in a single layer on a baking tray covered with baking paper.
6. Bake for 20 minutes, or until slightly crisp and coloured.

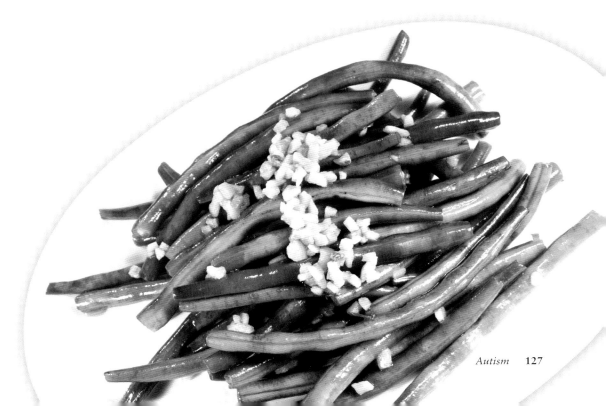

BANANA CASHEW & COCONUT MILK SMOOTHIE

INGREDIENTS

1 ripe banana (fresh or frozen for a thicker smoothie)

½ cup (125ml) cashew milk or almond milk

1 can organic, full fat coconut milk

½ tsp cinnamon

1 tsp honey or a few drops of Stevia to sweeten

METHOD

1. Blend all ingredients together and enjoy!

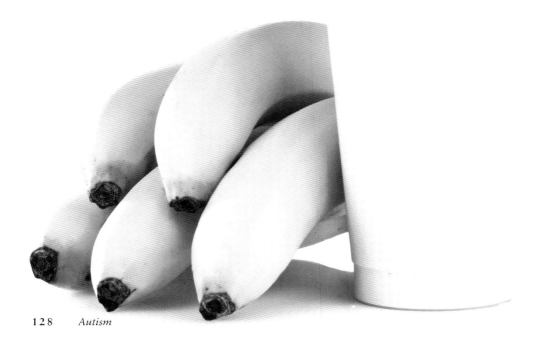